A Seminar

on

CURRENT TECHNICAL TOPICS

Presented at the

27th Annual Meeting of the

AMERICAN ASSOCIATION OF BLOOD BANKS

ANAHEIM, CALIFORNIA

November 11, 1974

Mention of specific commercial products or equipment by contributors to the American Association of Blood Banks' Seminar on Current Technical Topics does not represent an endorsement of such products by the American Association of Blood Banks, nor does it necessarily indicate a preference for those products over other similar competitive products.

Copyright © by American Association of Blood Banks 1974

All rights reserved. No part of this book may be reproduced or transmitted in any form or by any means, electronic or mechanical, including photocopying, recording or by any information storage and retrieval system, without permission in writing from the Publisher.

American Association of Blood Banks
Central Office. Suite 608
1828 L Street, N.W.
Washington, D.C. 20036

ISBN 0-914404-08-5

First Printing
Printed in the United States of America

 THE GUNTHORP-WARREN PRINTING COMPANY, CHICAGO

COMMITTEE ON TECHNICAL PROGRAM

RICHARD H. WALKER, M.D., Chairman
William Beaumont Hospital Blood Bank
Royal Oak, Michigan

ULA T. BLOCK, M.T.(ASCP)SBB
Touro Infirmary Blood Bank
New Orleans, Louisiana

MARY ANN GRALNICK M.T.(ASCP)SBB
Clinical Center Blood Bank
National Institutes of Health
Bethesda, Maryland

PAUL V. HOLLAND, M.D.
Clinical Center Blood Bank
National Institutes of Health
Bethesda, Maryland

DOUGLAS W. HUESTIS, M.D.
Department of Pathology
Arizona Medical Center
Tucson, Arizona

PETER D. ISSITT, F.I.M.L.T.
Paul I. Hoxworth Blood Center of
University of Cincinnati
Cincinnati, Ohio

BYRON A. MYHRE, M.D., Ph.D.
Harbor General Hospital
Torrance, California

JACOB NUSBACHER, M.D.
Rochester Regional Red Cross Blood Program
Rochester, New York

MARY BETH OLIVE, M.T.(ASCP)SBB
Blood Bank, University Hospital
Birmingham, Alabama

ARTHUR SIMMONS, L.C.S.L.T.
　Department of Pathology
　University Hospital
　Iowa City, Iowa

LOUISE WILSON WRIGHT, M.T.(ASCP)SBB
　Consultant
　Southwest Florida Blood Bank
　Tampa, Florida

PROGRAM PARTICIPANTS

ALTER, HARVEY J., M.D.—Chief, Immunology Section, Clinical Center Blood Bank, National Institutes of Health, Bethesda, Maryland

ASHCAVAI, MARY, M.T.(ASCP)—Supervisor, Clinical Laboratory, University of Southern California, John Wesley Hospital, Los Angeles, California

BLOCK, ULA T., M.T.(ASCP)SBB—Chief Technologist, Touro Infirmary Blood Bank, New Orleans, Louisiana

HUESTIS, DOUGLAS W., M.D.—Professor of Pathology, University of Arizona College of Medicine; Medical Director, Southern Arizona Red Cross Blood Center, Tucson, Arizona

McCULLOUGH, JEFFREY, M.D.—Associate Professor, Laboratory Medicine and Pathology and Director, Blood Bank, University of Minnesota Hospitals; Medical Director, St. Paul Regional Red Cross Blood Center, St. Paul, Minnesota

MAYER, KLAUS, M.D.—President, American Association of Blood Banks; Director, Hematology Laboratory, Memorial Hospital for Cancer and Allied Diseases, New York City; Clinical Associate Professor of Medicine, Cornell University Medical College

NUSBACHER, JACOB, M.D.—Medical Director, Rochester Regional Red Cross Blood Program; Assistant Professor of Medicine, University of Rochester, Rochester, New York

OBERMAN, HAROLD A., M.D.—Professor of Pathology and Medical Director, Blood Bank, University of Michigan Medical Center, Ann Arbor, Michigan

SCHMIDT, PAUL, J., M.D.—Chief, Blood Bank Department, Clinical Center, National Institutes of Health; Medical Director, Public Health Service, U. S. Department of Health, Education, and Welfare, Bethesda, Maryland

SLICHTER, SHERRILL J., M.D.—Assistant Director, King County Central Blood Bank; Assistant Professor in Medicine, University of Washington School of Medicine, Seattle, Washington

SOLIS, R. THOMAS, M.D.—Assistant Professor of Medicine, Baylor College of Medicine, Houston, Texas

WRIGHT, LOUISE WILSON, M.T.(ASCP)SBB—Consultant, Southwest Florida Blood Bank, Inc., Tampa, Florida

Program

PRECONVENTION SEMINAR
November 11, 1974

CURRENT TECHNICAL TOPICS

Ula T. Block, Moderator

8:55— 9:30 RADIOIMMUNOASSAY TESTS FOR HEPATITIS B SURFACE ANTIGEN: PROBLEMS, PRACTICALITIES AND PROMISES

Harvey J. Alter

9:30—10:00 HEPATITIS B ANTIGEN TESTING. OTHER METHODS AND INTERPRETATIONS

Mary Ashcavai

10:00—10:30 INTERMISSION

10:30—11:00 MICROEMBOLIZATION AND BLOOD TRANSFUSION

R. Thomas Solis

11:00—12:00 PRESENTATION OF THE EMILY COOLEY AWARD

Klaus Mayer

THE EMILY COOLEY LECTURE: TRANSFUSION IN HISTORICAL PERSPECTIVE

Paul J. Schmidt

Louise W. Wright, Moderator

2:00— 2:30 DISEASES TRANSMITTED BY BLOOD TRANSFUSION

Harold A. Oberman

2:30— 3:00 PREPARATION AND STORAGE OF PLATELET CONCENTRATES

Sherrill J. Slichter

3:00— 3:30   INTERMISSION

3:30— 4:00   GRANULOCYTE TRANSFUSION
             Jeffrey McCullough

4:00— 4:30   FRESH BLOOD: FACT AND FANCY
             Douglas W. Huestis

4:30— 5:15   FACULTY PANEL DISCUSSION
             AUDIENCE PARTICIPATION
             QUESTIONS AND ANSWERS
             Jacob Nusbacher, Moderator

THE EMILY COOLEY LECTURE

TODAY's lecture is the twelfth in a series of annual lectures in honor of Emily Cooley an outstanding medical technologist,
Emily Cooley was an attractive young woman reared in a distinguished family—her grandfather had been a Justice of the Supreme Court of Michigan and her father was a professor of pediatrics at Wayne University. She had been brought up to be an artist, or perhaps a writer, or simply to be a lady to preside over a civilized household like that of her mother. She had gone to a private girls' school, graduated from Vassar College, and taken a degree in landscaping. She gave up this promising career to tend the needs of her family. Her mother, a kindly, gracious woman, was often incapacitated by attacks of melancholia and her father, then about to retire, was ailing much of the time. Emily ran the household and was her father's companion, chauffeur, traveling aide, nurse, secretary and illustrator. It was she who made the beautiful drawings of blood films that appeared in Dr. Cooley's publications.

After the death of both of her parents, Emily, no longer young, had to find a career in which to earn a living. Having been so intimately connected with medicine, and hematology in particular, she chose medical technology. She took her training at Henry Ford Hospital and received a Master's Degree before she started work. When she was ready she naturally returned to the Children's Hospital where she so often had been a visitor in the laboratory with her father. She became the chief hematology technician, and was an excellent morphologist and the mainstay of that department. She was looked up to and beloved by her colleagues and happy in her work. Emily Cooley was not only a fine technologist and a dedicated worker in the laboratory but she was a warm, sensitive, intelligent and gracious human being. It is to her memory that this series of lectures is dedicated.

THE 1974 EMILY COOLEY LECTURER
Paul J. Schmidt, M.D.

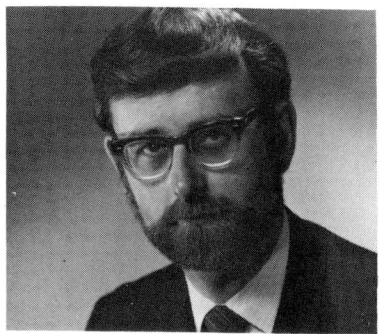

Dr. Paul J. Schmidt began a career in laboratory medicine when he came to the National Institutes of Health in 1954. His interest in blood dates back to 1948 when he began studies on the "Freezable Water of Blood" which was the title of his Master's thesis awarded by the Institute of Biophysics at St. Louis University. He continued the research while at the New York University-Bellevue Medical Center where he earned his M.D. in 1953.

His career in transfusion has been one of the application of research to practical hospital blood banking at the Clinical Center, the hospital of NIH. As the sole active survivor of the old Laboratory of Biologic Control and then a member of the Division of Biologics Standards of NIH, as well as the Standards Committee of the AABB, he has been involved also in many of the decisions which set the state of our art today.

For the past ten years, Dr. Schmidt has led a program of study of posttransfusion hepatitis, beginning with an assay of the prevalence of the disease after open heart surgery. Utilization of that model made possible definitive studies on the role of the commercial donor and the hepatitis antigens in our current knowledge of that disease.

In more than 80 published papers he has collaborated with a research team working on immunohematology, microbiology, transplantation, and blood component therapy; a team he gathered, trained and led.

Dr. Schmidt has been responsible for the training of many senior technologists and medical directors of blood banks and is Clinical Professor of Pathology at Georgetown University. He was Secretary General of the International Transfusion Congress held in Washington in 1972, and is currently the Chairman of the Scientific Program Committee of the AABB. He serves in an advisory capacity to the Blood Program of the American National Red Cross and other national organizations in hematology and clinical pathology. He was Assistant Chief of the Clinical Pathology Department at NIH from 1962 to 1964 and is certified by the American Board of Pathology both in Clinical Pathology and in Blood Banking.

In his research and literary endeavors, Dr. Schmidt is actively assisted by his wife, Louise, who is a medical librarian, and three children, Dan, Matt and Maria, all of whom have been seen at transfusion meetings for many years.

EMILY COOLEY LECTURERS

1963	E. Eric Muirhead, M.D.
1964	Scott N. Swisher, M.D.
1965	Wolf W. Zuelzer, M.D.
1966	Alexander S. Wiener, M.D.
1967	M. M. Strumia, M.D.
1968	Hugh Chaplin, Jr., M.D.
1969	Emanuel Hackel, Ph.D.
1970	Flemming Kissmeyer-Nielsen, M.D., Ph.D.
1971	Neva Martin Abelson, M.D.
1972	Bernard Pirofsky, M.D.
1973	Serafeim P. Masouredis, M.D.

Introduction

ALTHOUGH new red cell antigens and antibodies continue to be reported and the serology of the red cell is still under intensive investigation, the major activity in blood banking today is directed at improvement in other aspects of hemotherapy. The chapters in this book treat some of the areas of current special interest in providing a high quality and safe transfusion to meet special patient needs.

Some of the topics considered are controversial today, but of sufficient importance to warrant consideration. What is the best temperature at which one should store platelet concentrates—room temperature or 4 C? What is the best method to harvest granulocytes and when should they be used? Are granulocytes obtained from random unmatched donors of any value? Do significant increases in antibody titer to the cytomegalovirus following tranfusion indicate transmission of the virus or activation of a latent infection? What is fresh blood, and is the definition of fresh blood the same for all patients? What are microaggregates and are they of clinical significance in terms of cause and effect in producing pulmonary insufficiency following transfusion? What is the optimal method in terms of sensitivity, specificity and economy in testing blood donors for HB_sAg? Why do we still encounter many cases of posttransfusion hepatitis utilizing donor blood negative for HB_sAg? What lessons have we learned from the past? Our problems reflect the level of sophistication in hemotherapy as it is practiced today.

The questions posed above have not been finally resolved, but are under study. It appears likely that none of these questions will have simple answers and that the correct answers may well be determined by the many variables which go into each unique patient-transfusion situation.

R. H. Walker, M.D.

TABLE OF CONTENTS

	Page
Committee on Technical Program	i
Program Participants	iii
Program	iv
The Emily Cooley Lecture	vi
The 1974 Emily Cooley Lecturer	vii
Emily Cooley Lecturers	viii
Introduction	ix
RICHARD H. WALKER	
Radioimmunoassay Tests for Hepatitis B Surface Antigen: Problems, Practicalities, and Promises	1
HARVEY J. ALTER	
Hepatitis B Antigen Testing: Other Methods and Interpretations	13
MARY ASHCAVAI	
Microembolization and Blood Transfusion	31
R. THOMAS SOLIS	
The Emily Cooley Lecture: Transfusion in Historical Perspective	49
PAUL J. SCHMIDT	
Diseases Transmitted by Blood Transfusion	73
HAROLD A. OBERMAN	
Preparation and Storage of Platelet Concentrates	87
SHERRILL J. SLICHTER and LAURENCE A. HARKER	
Granulocyte Transfusion	95
JEFFREY MCCULLOUGH	
Fresh Blood: Fact and Fancy	117
DOUGLAS W. HUESTIS	

PROBLEMS, PRACTICALITIES, AND PROMISES
RADIOIMMUNOASSAY TESTS FOR HEPATITIS B SURFACE ANTIGEN:

Harvey J. Alter

SUBSEQUENT to the initial demonstration of Australia antigen (hepatitis B surface antigen, HB_sAg) utilizing the technique of agar gel diffusion, further increases in our understanding of type B hepatitis ("serum" hepatitis) and of the hepatitis B virus have been dependent upon a series of technologic advances. Progressively more sensitive tests for HB_sAg and for antibody to HB_sAg (anti-HB_s) have provided major insights into the frequency, distribution, mode of transmission and clinical significance of this antigenic marker. An evaluation of one such sensitive test for HB_sAg, radioimmunoassay, forms the basis for this report.

Relationship of HB_sAg to the Hepatitis B Virus

Before discussing specific assays, it is pertinent to review our current understanding of the relationship of HB_sAg to the hepatitis B virus (HBV). When HB_sAg was first associated with viral hepatitis, it was noted that HB_sAg-rich material contained 20 nm spherical virus-like particles and some associated tubular forms of similiar diameter.[4] These particles however, lacked internal complexity, could not be reproducibly shown to contain nucleic acid, could not be grown in tissue culture and generally did not fulfill the criteria for other known viruses. In 1970, using the technique of immune electron microscopy, Dane described a new particulate form associated with HB_sAg.[5] This Dane particle consists of an outer shell and an inner core, the latter with sufficient structural complexity to suggest that it is a true virus. HB_sAg has been shown to reside only on the outer shell and, hence, its current designation, hepatitis B surface antigen. The core lacks HB_sAg, but has its own antigenic determinant, now known as hepatitis B core antigen or HB_cAg. Recently, DNA polymerase, a virus-specific enzyme, has been localized within the core of the Dane particle (14), providing additional support that this particle represents the true hepatitis B virus.

Combining electron microscopic and fluorescent antibody observations,[3] it is now probable that the core of the Dane particle is produced in the nucleus of hepatocytes. Cores are then apparently released into the cytoplasm where they are enveloped by HB_sAg-containing coat material to form the complete hepatitis B virus. In addition, an enormous excess of HB$_s$Ag is produced in the cytoplasm and released unassembled into the blood stream where it circulates as the 20 nm spherical and tubular forms. Hence, the vast majority of antigen measured by tests for HB$_s$Ag represents incomplete virus which, by inference, is noninfectious. Epidemiologic studies, as well as serologic tests for HB$_s$Ag, have clearly distinguished hepatitis B virus ("serum") from hepatitis A virus ("infectious"), and have shown that hepatitis B virus infection is much more prevalent in our population than previously suspected. Transmission of HBV by routes other than "serum" probably accounts in large measure for the dissemination of this virus, although the exact modes of transmission are not clearly defined.

Comparison of Tests for HB$_s$Ag

Tests for HB$_s$Ag can be grouped into three major divisions based on relative sensitivity. The first, and for a long time, sole, test for HB$_s$Ag was double diffusion in agar (Ouchterlony, agar gel diffusion, AGD).[16] This is now considered the first generation test for HB$_s$Ag and provides the baseline against which the sensitivity of other tests is compared. The second generation of tests included complement fixation,[18] counterelectrophoresis (CEP),[9] hemagglutination inhibition,[23] and a variety of others. These tests were roughly equal in sensitivity and, on the average, 20 times more sensitive than AGD as based on comparative titers. The advent of radioimmunoassay tests for HB$_s$Ag[25] initiated the third generation of tests now characterized primarily by a solid phase radioimmunoassay,[15] and by reverse passive hemagglutination. These tests are approximately 100 times as sensitive as CEP and 2000 times as sensitive as AGD. This marked increase in sensitivity is not, however, reflected in a proportionate increase in the number of HB$_s$Ag-positive blood donors detected. The best current estimate is that RIA will detect 2 to 3 times as many HB$_s$Ag-positive donors as CEP.

Principles of Radioimmunoassay Tests

There have been two major types of radioimmunoassay (RIA) tests for HB$_s$Ag — the double antibody RIA (DA-RIA) and the solid phase RIA (SP-RIA), the principles of which are depicted in Figures 1 and 2. In DA-RIA (Figure 1), purified antigen is radio labelled and a known quantity is mixed with the sample to be tested. A limiting quantity of specific antibody is then added, establishing a competition for this antibody between the labelled antigen (AGN*) and any anti-

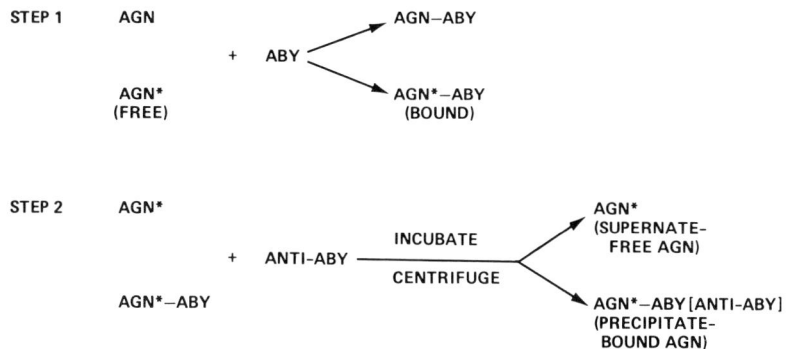

FIGURE 1: General principles of double antibody radioimmunoassay (see text for details). AGN = antigen; AGN* = radiolabelled antigen; ABY = antibody; AGN-ABY = antigen-antibody complex; Anti-ABY = antibody to immunoglobulin or to specific subclass of immunoglobulin. To relate this to radioimmunoassay for hepatitis B surface antigen (HBsAg), substitute HBsAg for AGN, ^{125}I-labelled HBsAg for AGN* and anti-HBs for antibody.

gen present in the sample. If no antigen is present in the sample, then most of the labelled antigen will combine with antibody to form an immune complex (bound, AGN*-ABY). Only a small amount of labelled antigen will remain free in solution. If, on the other hand, the sample contains the antigen, it will compete effectively with labelled antigen, and both labelled and unlabelled complexes will be formed. In this way, less of the labelled antigen will be in the complexed (bound) form and more will remain free. Indeed, the ratio of bound to free radio labelled antigen will be directly proportional to the amount of competing antigen in the sample. In order to determine how much is bound and how much is free, a second step is introduced into the procedure (Figure 1, step 2). Antibody to immunoglobulin or to one specific class of immunoglobulin is added to the reaction mixture. This will precipitate labelled antigen which is bound to antibody, but will leave unbound antigen in the supernate. One can then determine radioactive counts in the supernate and/or the precipitate to establish a bound-to-free ratio. A standard curve is established which relates the bound/free ratio to known quantities of antigen, and in this way the amount of antigen in an unknown sample can be established.

The DA-RIA remains the standard method for most radioimmunoassays in clinical medicine, and some feel it is the most sensitive RIA for detecting HB$_s$Ag.[13] However, a simpler and more practical method[15] has become the standard RIA employed by blood banks for HB$_s$Ag testing. This solid phase RIA is depicted in Figure 2. Here, unlabelled antibody to HB$_s$Ag (anti-HB$_s$) is attached to a solid support usually

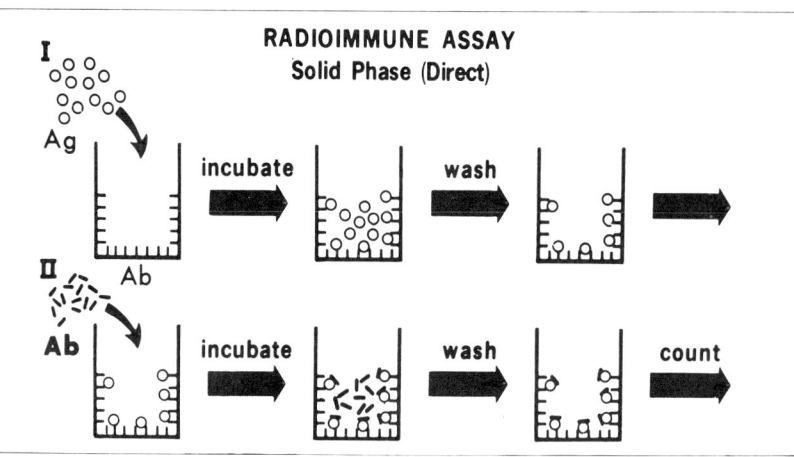

FIGURE 2: General principles of solid phase radioimmunoassay for hepatitis B surface antigen (HB$_s$Ag). See text for details. Unlabelled antibody to HB$_s$Ag (anti-HB$_s$) is attached to a polystyrene tube as indicated by short perpendicular lines in the first diagram. HB$_s$Ag is indicated by the open circles and in stage I HB$_s$Ag attaches to anti-HB$_s$ on the tube. In stage II ^{125}I-labelled anti-HB$_s$ is added as indicated by the thick black rods. Labelled anti-HB$_s$ attaches to HB$_s$Ag and is then counted. Counts are compared with a negative control.

(Reprinted with permission of Dr. Lacy R. Overby from a workshop on radioimmunoassay sponsored by Abbott Laboratories.)

either a polystyrene tube, a microtiter plate,[19] or a bead. The solid support with its attached anti-HB$_s$ is then immersed in the sample to be tested followed by an appropriate incubation period. If HB$_s$Ag is present, it will attach to the anti-HB$_s$, and hence adhere to the tube while other proteins will be washed out. In the second phase of this test, ^{125}I-labelled anti-HB$_s$ is added. If HB$_s$Ag was present in the original sample, some of its antigenic sites will have attached to unlabelled antibody on the solid support; other antigenic sites, however, will be available to attach to the ^{125}I-labelled antibody, thus forming a sandwich of labelled antibody - antigen - unlabelled antibody. In the presence of HB$_s$Ag, the labelled antibody will remain firmly adherent to the tube. In the absence of HB$_s$Ag, labelled antibody will wash out of the tube during the final washing procedure. The radioactivity in the tube is then counted and the number of counts is roughly proportional to the amount of antigen present in the original sample. Semi-quantitation is achieved by doing repetitive determinations (usually eight) on a sample known to lack HB_sAg. The mean of these determinations is used as the negative baseline, and the counts in each unknown sample are compared with this negative control. A cutoff value of 2.1 has been established such that a sample which has more than 2.1 times the radioactive counts of the negative control is considered HB_sAg-positive. The higher the ratio of sample counts to control counts, the more antigen present, although this relationship is not strictly quantitative. Since SP-RIA (Ausria), represents the only currently licensed RIA for HB_sAg, the remainder of this discussion will focus on this specific procedure.

Sensitivity of Solid Phase-RIA

There are many ways to assess the relative sensitivity of various test methods. Most commonly employed is the performance of serial dilutions and determination of end-point titers. Employing this method, we have found that SP-RIA could detect HB_sAg at dilutions 75 times that which could be detected by CEP, the most commonly used second generation test.[1] In a panel distributed to several laboratories by the National Heart and Lung Institute (NHLI), SP-RIA achieved average titers 20 times that of the second generation tests.[20] The increased sensitivity of SP-RIA can also be demonstrated using undiluted sera; CEP-positive sera are, almost universally, also RIA-positive. In contrast, the finding of RIA-positive, CEP-negative sera is not unusual. This has been clearly demonstrated by proficiency panels distributed by AABB, the Bureau of Biologics, and the NHLI. The increased sensitivity of SP-RIA over CEP is also demonstrated in patients presenting with acute hepatitis, in animals experimentally infected with HB_sAg, and in patients recovering from HB_sAg-positive hepatitis where it can be shown that antigen is detectable for weeks to months longer by SP-RIA than by CEP.[1]

Specificity of SP-RIA

Non-specificity has in the past been a major problem in the SP-RIA test and, indeed, initial claims that it would detect 10-20 times as many HB_sAg-positive blood donors as CEP were based on the detection of false positive reactions. Non-specificity in the SP-RIA was first described by Sgouris[22] who found that certain laboratory workers had anti-guinea pig antibodies capable of reacting with the guinea pig-derived anti-HB$_s$ used in the Ausria test. This was initially considered an isolated problem confined to guinea pig handlers, but subsequently, four independent laboratories demonstrated rates of non-specific reactions among normal blood donors ranging from 75 to 90%.[1, 12, 17, 24] On the average, about half the non-specificity was due to antibodies present in normal serum which were capable of reacting with guinea pig proteins utilized as reagents in the Ausria test. The cause of the other non-specific reactions could not be determined. This would appear to be an inordinate and unacceptable degree of non-specificity. However, it has subsequently been shown that the high degree of non-specificity was related to certain production lots of Ausria, and that residual non-specificity could be greatly reduced by modifications in the Ausria system. These modifications include: (1) incorporation of normal guinea pig serum into the ^{125}I-anti-HB$_s$ reagent guinea pig so as to neutralize non-specific human antibody capable of crossreacting with guinea pig anti-HB$_s$; (2) performance of the test at 45 C, speeding the reaction and favoring true reactivity; (3) the use of one species of antibody to coat the tube (e.g. guinea pig) and another species to serve as labelled reagent (e.g. human). The first two modifications have been incorporated into the standard Ausria test and have greatly reduced non-specificity. The third modification now incorporated into the Ausria II test appears to reduce non-specific reactions to under 1%.

Non-specificity is thus no longer a significant problem in this assay. It is, however, essential that the potential for non-specific reactions be considered whenever an Ausria-positive, CEP-negative result occurs. The implications of falsely labelling an individual as HB$_s$Ag-positive are considerable, and no donor or patient should be so labelled until appropriate specificity testing is complete. The theoretical basis for such specificity testing is simple. If the positive result is due to interaction between HB$_s$Ag and radiolabelled anti-HB$_s$, i.e. a true positive, then the reaction can be neutralized by incubating the HB$_s$Ag with unlabelled human anti-HB$_s$ prior to incubation with the standard reagent. The "cold" antibody will block specific antigenic sites on the HB$_s$Ag containing particle, and prevent its subsequent reaction with labelled anti-HB$_s$. A reduction in radioactive counts of greater than 50% between the neutralized and standard reaction is considered evidence of specificity. If, on the other hand, reactivity was due to anti-guinea pig antibody or other non-specific effects, radioactive counts will not be significantly diminished by prior incubation with unlabelled human anti-HB$_s$. To reiterate, because the psychologic, sociologic and economic consequences of labelling a donor as HB$_s$Ag-positive may be far-reaching, it is essential that the specificity of RIA-positive, CEP-negative reactions be determined. Such specificity testing is uncomplicated and can be readily incorporated into the standard test procedure.

One last point regarding specificity must be raised. Some studies of posttransfusion hepatitis performed at a time when non-specificity was a major problem, demonstrated a poor correlation between SP-RIA positivity and subsequent recipient infectivity. However, since these studies did not include specificity testing, and since at that time as much as 80% of SP-RIA positives may have been false positives, the poor correlation was to have been anticipated. When specificity is taken into account, as will be shown in the table on page 10, the correlation with infectivity is quite good.

Advantages and Disadvantages of RIA Tests

The major advantage of RIA tests over second generation tests is, of course, their increased sensitivity. However, another significant advantage is their inherent objectivity. Proficiency panels distributed by AABB and the Bureau of Biologics have shown that weakly positive CEP reactions are consistently missed by the average technologist due to inability to read faint precipitin lines. These same weak reactions, subject to intepretive error in CEP, would produce relatively high counts by RIA, and would be unequivocally positive even to inexperienced personnel. Thus, not only is CEP less sensitive than RIA, but reader error exaggerates this insensitivity even further. The same may be true for any test which has a subjective endpoint and might include reversed passive hemagglutination assays as well. In essence, whatever the absolute sensitivity of a given procedure, this sensitivity will be diminished by interpretive error in proportion to the subjectivity of the end point. Such error needlessly endangers the blood recipient and subjects the recipient to a hepatitis risk which could be largely avoided by RIA. Despite these important benefits of RIA, there are several disadvantages of such a test system. The major disadvantages are high cost and prolonged test time. RIA tests require a large initial investment by the blood bank to purchase a gamma scintillation detector, unless such a machine can be shared with an existing facility in the hospital. In addition to this initial cost, RIA for HB$_s$Ag requires a high per test expenditure. It is very difficult, however, to assess cost in the abstract. The cost of a test must be weighed against its benefits to the patient; there are many ethical as well as practical considerations which enter into the calculation of cost-benefit ratios related to a radioimmunoassay test whose objective is to reduce posttransfusion hepatitis. What is the cost of a serious case of hepatitis? What is the price of death due to hepatitis? Does one consider cost to society, cost to the family, or cost to the patient? For the most part, these costs are incalculable. It would seem that if a test can be proven to reduce posttransfusion hepatitis to a greater extent than any other available test, then its cost must be incurred. As will be shown below, it is clear that SP-RIA is effective in reducing type B posttransfusion hepatitis as compared to CEP. Similar data comparing SP-RIA and RPH are not available at the time of this writing. If RPH can be proven equally effective at lesser cost, then this would strongly weigh in its favor. If, however, RPH or any other test that might be developed, is not comparable to RIA in its ability to prevent type B posttransfusion hepatitis, then it should not be adopted no matter what its financial and practical benefits.

The time required for SP-RIA has been greatly reduced by performing the test at 45 C rather than at room temperature. This temperature speeds the reaction time without reducing sensitivity and, as previously stated, it has the added benefit of reducing non-specificity. However, even at 45 C, the test requires 3 hours of incubation time plus additional time for sample preparation, washing, and counting. In practical terms, this means that blood drawn one day is not ready for distribution until the following morning. It also usually means employment of at least one additional person to perform this procedure in the evening. A more rapid test would be of great advantage if it could be achieved without a loss in sensitivity. The potential for this is greater for RPH than for further modification in SP-RIA. However, again, the efficacy of such a rapid system in preventing type B posttransfusion hepatitis would have to be proven.

In performing RIA tests (as well as others) one can get positive results which are not reproducible, or one can get reproducible results which are, none the less, non-specific, i.e. false positives. Modifications in SP-RIA have reduced the latter to an acceptable minimum and, as mentioned, every reproducible positive result must undergo specificity testing before being reported. The frequency of non-repeatable results by the heat method appears to be less than 1%, a nuisance requiring temporary quarantine of some blood units, but not a major problem. The number of non-reproducible results varies from run to run as some tests appear to be overly "sensitive." We have found it useful to incorporate a standard curve each day as an index of the sensitivity of that assay and as a means of comparing test results from day to day. This provides better quality control than simply running the one positive control sample provided.

Impact of RIA Tests on Posttransfusion Hepatitis

There is little doubt that screening donors by CEP has reduced the frequency of type B posttransfusion hepatitis.[2, 10, 21] It has, however, been estimated that CEP would prevent no more than 25% of total PTH.[10] The reasons for this low estimate are now increasingly clear. Prospective studies of PTH utilizing CEP-tested, voluntary donor blood have demonstrated that PTH is due to at least two viral agents,[2] and current data indicate that an increasing proportion of posttransfusion hepatitis cases are serologically unrelated to the hepatitis B virus. The etiology of these "Non-B" hepatitis cases has not been established. Using a newly described test for antibody to hepatitis virus A,[6] we have shown that "Non-B" hepatitis is serologically unrelated to virus A.[7] In addition, most of these cases do not demonstrate a serologic response to CMV or EB virus. There is, thus, increasing suspicion that there is at least one additional, heretofore unrecognized, human hepatitis virus (type C?).

It is important to emphasize that no matter how sensitive tests for HB_sAg become, they will only be effective in preventing type B hepatitis and will have no impact on hepatitis due to other viral agents. Extrapolation from available data on recipients of CEP-negative, voluntary donor blood suggests that even the ultimate test for HB_sAg will prevent no more than 50%, and perhaps as low as 25%, of total posttransfusion hepatitis. Counterbalancing this pessimistic prediction, however, is the fact that acute type B hepatitis seems to be more severe than that due to other viral agents. Thus, while screening tests for HB_sAg will prevent only a portion of total hepatitis, they may prevent the majority of overt serious illness. It is probable that chronic sequelae of hepatitis are also more common and more severe after type B infection, but this has not been proved. The prevention of type B hepatitis may thus have benefits to the patient disproportionate to its actual frequency in the recipient population.

All prospective studies of PTH have indicated that some type B hepatitis continues to occur despite the exclusion of HB_sAg-positive donors detectable by CEP. How effective would RIA tests be in detecting these low-grade carriers of HBV and in preventing residual type B hepatitis infection? Published studies relating RIA to prevention of overt type B hepatitis in recipients of CEP-negative blood are summarized in the Table. In addition, this table includes unpublished data from our laboratory indicating that 3 out of 4 cases of type B hepatitis following CEP-negative blood could have been prevented if donors had initially been screened by SP-RIA. The data of Giorgini and Hollinger demonstrate the efficacy of DA-RIA and the data of Gocke indicate that 5 of 18 episodes of type B hepatitis might have been prevented if SP-RIA rather than CEP had been used for donor screening. There are now several additional studies in progress. Personal communications from Dr. Richard Aach of the Barnes-Wohl hospital in St. Louis, Dr. Alfred Prince of the New York Blood Center, and Dr. Gary Gitnick of the University of California at Los Angeles all indicate that most, but not all, of type B posttransfusion hepatitis could be prevented if the SP-RIA was routinely employed for HB_sAg testing of blood donors.

TABLE

Results of Retrospective Testing by RIA of CEP-Negative Donors Implicated in Type B Posttransfusion Hepatitis.

Author	Reference	Method	# Type B Hepatitis	# In Which RIA-Positive Donor Detected
Giorgini	8	DA-RIA	5	5
Gocke	11	SP-RIA	18	5
Hollinger	13	DA-RIA	2	2
		SP-RIA	2	0
Alter	Unpublished	SP-RIA	4	3

Summary

The data presented strongly indicate the need to replace CEP with a test of greater sensitivity and greater objectivity. It is clear that RIA-positive, CEP-negative donors exist and that their blood is capable of transmitting overt type B hepatitis. Although double antibody RIA may be the most sensitive of current tests, it is not practicable for routine utilization by blood banks. The only licensed third generation methods at present are solid phase-RIA (SP-RIA) and reversed passive hemagglutination (RPH). In our limited experience, SP-RIA is more sensitive than RPH, but more extensive comparisons of these two methods and of their impact on type B posttransfusion hepatitis (PTH) is required. It is also clear at present that third generation tests will not prevent all of type B hepatitis, and that at least half, and perhaps up to 80%, of PTH is now unrelated to the hepatitis B virus. Thus, the total prevention of PTH will have to depend upon the development of serologic tests for other involved virologic agents as well as further refinements in testing for HB_sAg. Alternately, methods to inactive or remove virus from donor blood, or methods to immunize the recipient will have to be developed. Such measures would be independent of testing. Of those measures currently available, it is mandatory that, as soon as possible, we: (1) totally exclude commercial blood donors and, (2) adopt a third generation test to supplant CEP for routine donor screening.

REFERENCES

1. Alter H, Holland PV, Purcell RH, et al: The Ausria test: critical evaluation of sensitivity and specificity. *Blood* **42**:947, 1973.
2. Alter HJ, Holland PV, Purcell RH, et al: Posttransfusion hepatitis after exclusion of commercial and hepatitis-B-antigen-positive donors. *Ann. Intern. Med.* **77**:691, 1972.
3. Barker LF, Chisari FV, McGrath PP, et al: Transmission of type B viral hepatitis to chimpanzees. *J. Infectious Diseases* **127**:648, 1973.
4. Bayer ME, Blumberg BS, Werner B: Particles associated with Australia antigen in the sera of patients with leukemia, Down's syndrome and hepatitis. *Nature* **218**:1057, 1968.
5. Dane DS, Cameron CH, Briggs M: Virus-like particles in serum of patients with Australia-antigen-associated hepatitis. *Lancet* **1**:695, 1970.
6. Feinstone SM, Kapikian AZ, Purcell RH: Hepatitis A: Detection by immune electron microscopsy of a virus-like antigen associated with acute illness. *Science* **182**:1026, 1973.
7. Feinstone SM, Alter HJ, Purcell RH: In preparation.
8. Giorgini GL, Hollinger FB, Leduc L, et al: Radioimmunoassay detection of hepatitis type B antigen. *JAMA* **222**:1514, 1972.
9. Gocke DJ, Howe C: Rapid detection of Australia antigen by counterelectrophoresis. *J. Immunology* **104**:1031, 1970.
10. Gocke, DJ, Greenberg HB, Kavey NB: Correlation of Australia antigen with posttransfusion hepatitis. *JAMA* **212**:877, 1970.
11. Gocke DJ, Kachani ZF: Evaluation of a new agglutination-flocculation test for the prevention of type B posttransfusion hepatitis

(abstract). Presented at 26th Annual Meeting American Association of Blood Banks, Bal Harbour, Florida, 1973.

12. Goldfield M: Annual progress report June 1, 1972 to July 1, 1973 to the Bureau of Biologics, FDA, Contract NIH-DBS-70-2026.

13. Hollinger FB, Werch J, Melnick JL: A prospective study indicating that double-antibody radioimmunoassay reduces the incidence of post-transfusion hepatitis B. *New Eng. J. Med.* **290**:1104, 1974.

14. Kaplan PM, Greenman RL, Gerin JL, et al: DNA polymerase associated with human hepatitis B antigen. *J. Virology* **12**:995, 1973.

15. Ling CA, Overby LR: Prevalence of hepatitis B virus antigen as revealed by direct radioimmune assay with I^{-125} antibody. *J. Immunology* **109**:834, 1972.

16. Prince AM: An antigen detected in the blood during the incubation period of serum hepatitis. *Proc. Natl. Acad. Sci. USA* **60**:814, 1968.

17. Prince AM, Brotman B, Joss D, et al: The specificity of this direct solid phase radioimmunoassay for detection of hepatitis B antigen. *Lancet* **1**:1346, 1973.

18. Purcell RH, Holland PV, Walsh JH, et al: A complement-fixation test for measuring Australia antigen and antibody. *J. Infectious Diseases* **120**:383, 1969.

19. Purcell RH, Wong DC, Alter HJ, et al: A microtiter solid-phase radioimmunoassay for hepatitis B antigen. *J. Appl. Microbiol.* **26**:478, 1973.

20. Roche JK, Stengle JM: Comparison of the sensitivities of the newer detection systems for hepatitis B antigen. *Transfusion* **13**:258, 1973.

21. Senior JR, Goeser E, Dahlke M, et al: Reduction in post-transfusion hepatitis after rejection of donor blood containing Australia antigen (abstract). *Gastroenterology* **60**:752, 1971.

22. Sgouris JT: Limitations of the radioimmunoassay for hepatitis B antigen. *New Eng. J. Med.* **288**:160, 1973.

23. Vyas, GN, Shulman NR: Hemagglutination assay for antigen and antibody associated with viral hepatitis. *Science* **170**:332, 1970.

24. Vyas GN, Adelberg SG, Perkins HA, et al: Non-specificity of hepatitis B antigen detected with iodine - 125 - labelled antibody. *Science* **182**:1368, 1973.

25. Walsh JH, Yalow R, Berson SA: Detection of Australia antigen and antibody by means of radioimmunoassay techniques. *J. Infectious Diseases* **121**:550, 1970.

HEPATITIS B ANTIGEN TESTING
OTHER METHODS AND INTERPRETATIONS
Mary Ashcavai

I. Hepatitis B (Surface) Antigen Testing

THE current techniques of testing for hepatitis B antigen (HB_sAg) cover a wide range of sensitivity. Differences in specific applications as well as relative sensitivity, cost and time utilized in the procedure influence the selection of method. The basic methods include antigen-antibody precipitation in agar, complement fixation (CF), hemagglutination inhibition (HAI), reversed passive hemagglutination (RPHA) and radioimmunoassay (RIA). The major varieties of agar precipitation are agar gel diffusion (AGD), rheophoresis (RHEO), and counterelectrophoresis (CEP). Many comparison studies have shown AGD to be the least sensitive and RIA the most sensitive of the commercially available tests. RHEO, CEP and CF are of approximately equal sensitivity while HAI and RPHA have greater sensitivity.[3, 16, 23] Accordingly, the more common tests listed in increasing order of sensitivity would appear as follows:

1. AGD
2. RHEO, CEP and CF
3. HAI
4. RPHA
5. RIA

Although the RIA method is the most sensitive method, there will be many laboratories still using one or more of the other less sensitive methods for various reasons, such as speed and economy in screening large numbers of sera, convenience when testing a small number of sera, back-up or alternate method, simultaneous testing of HB_sAg and anti-HB_sAg, confirmation of positive HB_sAg and anti HB_sAg, subtyping, etc.

This is a brief overview of the principles, advantages, disadvantages, pitfalls and interpretation of these methods.

1. **Agar gel diffusion (AGD)**

    a. *Principle*

    When HB_sAg and its specific antibody diffuse toward each other in an agar gel, a precipitin line will form at the point of optimal relative concentrations. Although AGD is slower and less sensitive than other methods for detecting HB_sAg, it has been valuable as a confirmatory test for sera shown to be HB_sAg positive by other methods.[2, 3, 21, 24] When concentrated serum is used for AGD, most positive reactions detected by the more sensitive methods can be confirmed. At our liver unit, an average of 68 patients are admitted per month with the diagnosis of acute viral hepatitis. Forty-eight percent have HB_sAg in their sera detectable by RIA. Of those positive sera, 94% can be confirmed by AGD using concentrated serum. However, during subsiding stages of viral hepatitis when antigen titers drop, AGD confirmation is not possible in as high a percentage.

The well pattern most frequently used for AGD is six wells arranged around a central one. Anti-HB_sAg is placed in the center well and HB_sAg positive control serum is placed in two opposite peripheral wells, 1 and 4 (Figure 1). The four remaining wells are used for

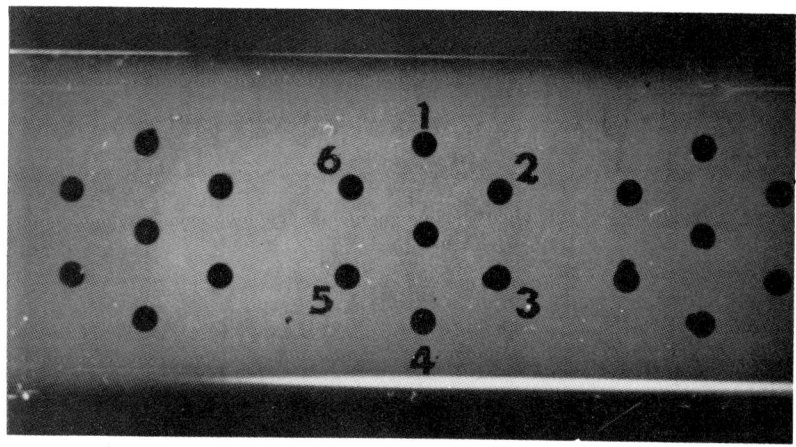

FIGURE 1: Pattern of wells commonly used for AGD. Each hexagonal set has control HB:Ag in wells 1 and 4, anti HB:Ag in the center and test serum in wells 2, 3, 5 and 6.

test sera. The placement of test wells adjacent to known positive antigen not only allows lines of identity for form but also results in a phenomenon that is referred to as an "enhancement" effect because the strongly reactive serum increases the visibility of the precipitation arc of an adjacent weakly reactive HB_sAg.[25] The pattern shown also allows a serum to be assayed for HB_sAg and anti-HB_sAg simultaneously since each test serum specimen is in apposition to both a well containing HB_sAg and a well containing anti-HB_sAg.

A precipitin line will form between the positive antigen controls in wells 1 and 4 and the center well. Strongly antigenic sera will show precipitin lines in less than 24 hours, most weakly antigenic sera will show precipitin lines in 2-3 days, while an occasional one will be seen after 6 days of incubation. When testing a weak antigen, the longer incubation time is required to allow the antibody which is in excess to diffuse into the agar until it reaches an optimal concentration relative to that of HB_sAg. Only then does precipitation occur since excess antibody results in soluble complexes. Concentration of weakly antigenic sera with polyacrilamide gel (Lyphogel®)[2,3] or Minicon-S®[3] before testing by AGD will shorten the incubation time.

When a precipitin line forms between a test well and the center well, the line must show identity with that of the control to be considered positive and specific (Figure 2). Branching or spurring of precipitin lines will occur when adjacent antigens are partially identical (Figure 3) (see *antigenic subtyping* under part b of Rheophoresis). False positive or nonspecific reactions are seen as precipitin lines which cross the control arc (Figure 4).

Antibody to HB_sAg is demonstrated by a precipitin line between the test well and the positive control forming a line of identity with the positive control (Figure 5).

b. *Advantages and disadvantages*

The advantages of AGD have been outlined above. There are certain obvious disadvantages.

Weakly antigenic specimens require a long incubation period (up to 7 days) to develop precipitin lines. Spurring or branching and crossing of precipitin lines usually require longer than overnight incubation to become visible. For this reason all positive AGD confirmation tests should be reread the day after the initial positive reading before they are discarded.

The accuracy and reliability of the AGD test is dependent upon careful reading of the reactions. This is best done with a small lamp in a darkened or dimly lit room. The slides are best viewed against a dull, dark background, directing the edge of the light beam toward the edge of the slide, while titling and slightly rotating the slide for maximum refractility of the precipitin arcs. Faint precipitin lines can be missed if the slides are read without manipulation. A magnifying glass may be helpful. Concentration of the sera will allow visualization of some serum reactions which might otherwise be missed (Figure 6A, B).

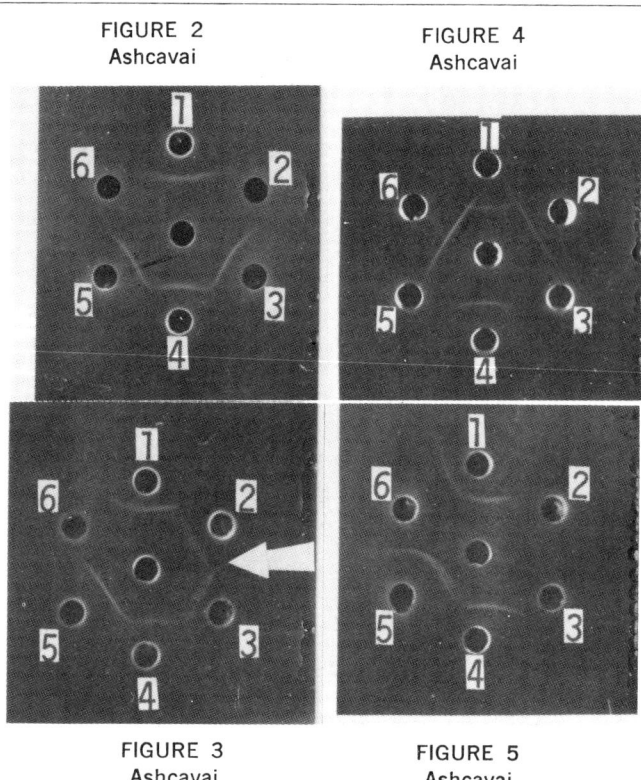

FIGURE 2
Ashcavai

FIGURE 4
Ashcavai

FIGURE 3
Ashcavai

FIGURE 5
Ashcavai

FIGURE 2: AGD showing HB$_s$Ag control in top (1) and bottom (4) wells with sera in wells 3 and 5 showing lines of identity with 4 control.

FIGURE 3: AGD with control HB$_s$AG in top (1) and bottom (4) wells and with positive sera in wells 2, 3 and 5. There is spurring indicating partial identity, between the precipitation arcs of sera in wells 2 and 3 (arrow).

FIGURE 4: In this pattern the AGD shows false positive reactions in wells 2 and 6 crossing that of HB$_s$Ag control arc in well 1.

FIGURE 5: Antibody can be detected on AGD as shown. Wells 1 and 4 are HB$_s$Ag control, 5 contains a serum specimen positive for HB$_s$Ag with line of identity to control, well 6 contains an antibody with arc between 6 and 1, and between 5 and 6, both forming lines of identity with the precipitation arcs of the adjacent wells.

2. **Rheophoresis**

a. *Principle*

Rheophoresis, rheo (flow or current) + phoresis (being borne), is an improved AGD.[14, 20] Antigen specimens placed in the peripheral

16

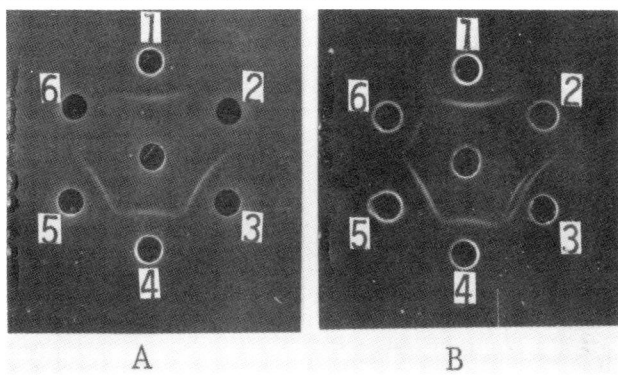

FIGURE 6: In 6A unconcentrated serum specimens show positive reactions with lines of identity in wells #3 and 5. Note that a fuzzy area at most is visible in well #6. In 6B the same serum specimens have been concentrated 10-fold with polyacrilamide gel. Note that the positive reaction in well #6 is readily apparent, and that the reaction of well #3 shows a double arc with lines of identity.

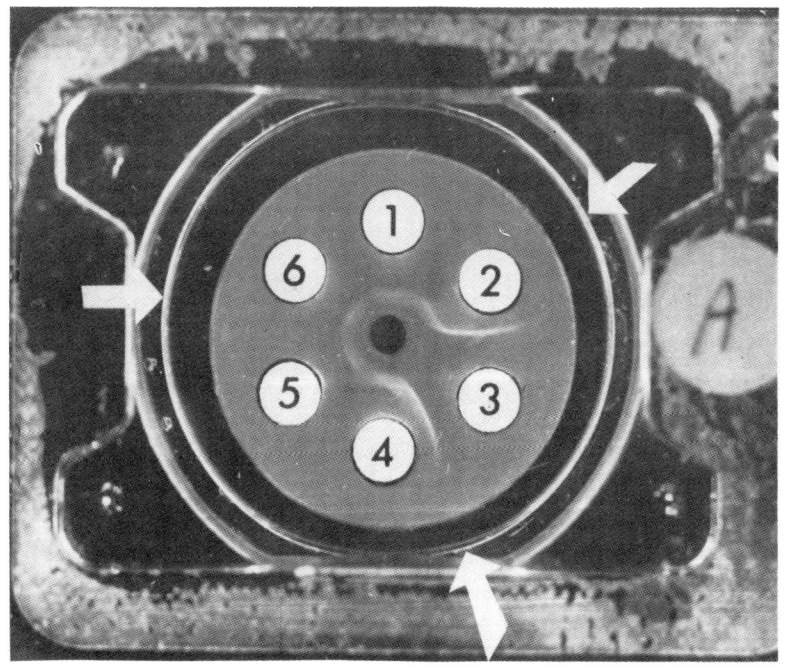

FIGURE 7: Rheophoresis with a round agar mound surrounded by a moat filled with buffer (arrows). Note the fuzzy precipitation arc when the antigen is quite strong. Well #3 contains antibody.

17

wells of a hexagonal test pattern are induced to flow only towards the central antibody well instead of radially. This is accomplished by the formation of a circular moat around the hexagonal pattern (Figure 7). Buffer is placed in the moat and the agar plate is covered by a plastic lid with a hole overlying the central antibody well. This promotes evaporation from the agar in the center, resulting in a flow of liquid within the agar from the peripheral moat towards the center carrying with it sera from the peripheral wells. Greater concentrations of the sera are delivered to the antibody by the prevention of radial diffusion.

b. *Advantages and disadvantages*

The sensitivity of this technique is at least comparable to CEP which makes it a practical method of choice for the laboratory that performs a few HB_sAg tests per day. It is to be preferred over AGD for confirmation of positives detected by other methods because the incubation time is greatly shortened for very weak positives (3 days instead of 7) as a result of the concentrating effect. The incubation time may be further shortened if the specimens are first concentrated 5-10 fold (by Lyphogel® or Minicon-S®) before testing. On the other

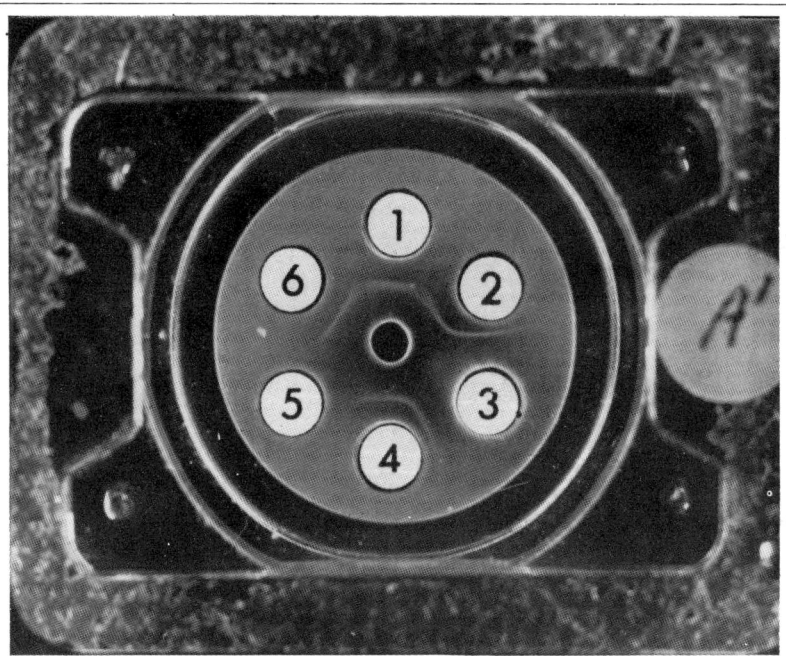

FIGURE 8: Note the sharp precipitation arcs on dilution of strongly reactive serum.

hand, a serum with a very high titer of HB_sAg may appear as a somewhat fuzzy arc very close to the central antibody well (Figure 7). When rheophoresis is to be used to establish lines of identity of positive sera, those identified as strongly reactive by the screening technique (CEP, CF, HAI) will have sharpened lines of identity if they are diluted 1:4 or 1:8 with saline before testing (Figure 8).

Specimens with very weak reactions by CEP, CF, or HAI which are negative by rheophoresis after two days of incubation sometimes will form precipitin lines by filling only the particular specimen well with saline or buffer every 2 to 3 hours during the day and incubating the plate overnight at room temperature.

Antigenic subtyping can be highly successful using rheophoresis.[20] There seems to be at least one group specific antigen, referred to as *a*, present in all HB_sAg particles, with at least several additional determinants; the most studied are *ad* and *ay*. The *d* and *y* determinants are thought to be alleles as they do not coexist.[18] Allelic subtypes *aw* and *ar*

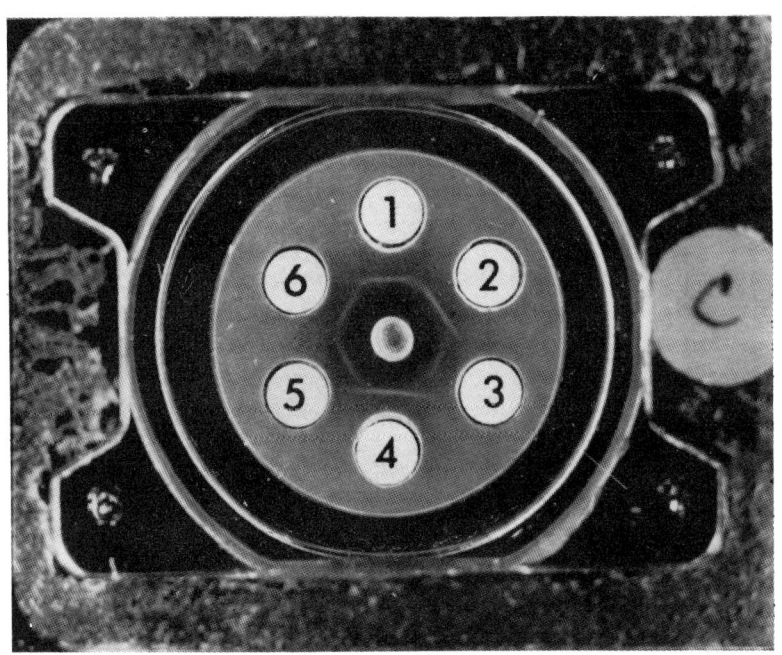

FIGURE 9: Rheophoresis used for subtyping. The antisera is anti-**ad**, whereas wells 3, 5 and 6, which are subtype **ay**, form arcs of partial identity.

have been studied less extensively. Subtype *ar* occurs predominantly in the Orient, *aw* in the rest of the world.[19] When antigen subtype *ad* is placed next to antigen subtype *ay* and diffused against anti-ad, a line of partial identity or spur will be formed by the precipitin arcs (Figure 9). The formation of a spur is sharpened when the titers of antigens used are low and of approximately equal level.

c. *Pitfalls*

Specimens with very high titers of HB_sAg will form fuzzy arcs close to the antibody well. These specimens should be diluted and the test repeated to show definite lines of identity with positive controls. An

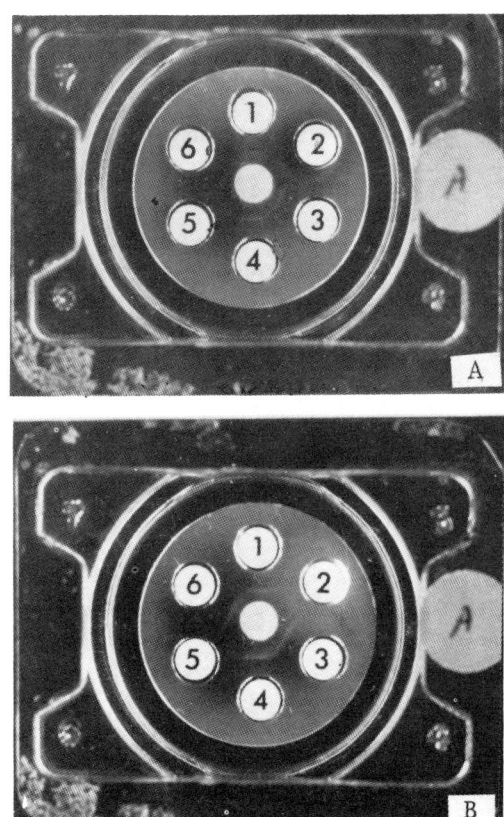

FIGURE 10: The fuzzy precipitation arcs of strong antigen (A) with the nonspecific reaction against well #2 can be remedied by adding buffer to the test wells every 2-3 hours (B).

occasional specimen will react non-specifically against other sera (Figure 10A) or against the agar by forming a hazy halo. Lipemic sera may appear the same way. This can usually be remedied by filling the particular test well with buffer or saline every 2 to 3 hours during the day and incubating the plates overnight at room temperature (Figure 10B).

One problem occasionally encountered with commercially available rheophoresis plates is the difficulty in removing the plastic ring which forms the moat without tearing the agar. The agar seems to be attached firmly to the plastic ring and must be separated with a sharp thin blade or scalpel before the ring can be gently removed. If the segment of agar between two test wells should tear, the plate may still be used if buffer does not appear in any of the wells when the moat is filled with buffer. The wells adjacent to the tear may be used for testing only if the same test sample or control is placed in both wells.

The above problem is eliminated when making your own rheophoresis plates by coating the plastic rings with a very thin film of mineral oil. Simply place 20 to 30 rings in a small beaker or pint size container, fill the container with hot tap water to just below the level of the rings, add one drop of mineral oil, cover the container and shake it up and down vigorously for a few seconds. Drain and rinse once with distilled water. The rings may be used directly or stored for later use.

3. Counterelectrophoresis (CEP)

a. *Principle*

If electrophoresis of serum specimens is undertaken in an alkaline medium, HB_sAg moves in the alpha 1 globulin range towards the anode while anti-HB_sAg moves in the opposite direction in the gamma fraction towards the cathode. When HB_sAg and anti-HB_sAg are properly placed in separate wells in the same plane with the antibody between the anode and the antigen, the two will move toward each other, meet, and form a precipitin line.[22] Anti-HB_sAg and HB_sAg may both be tested for concurrently in a serum specimen if three wells are placed in a row, test serum in the center, anti-HB_sAg on the anode side and control HB_sAg on the cathode side. A precipitin line forming between the known HB_sAg and the test serum indicates a probable anti-HB_sAg in the test serum, whereas a precipitation line between test specimen, and the anti-HB$_s$Ag well is presumptive evidence of HB$_s$Ag in serum (Figure 11).[3]

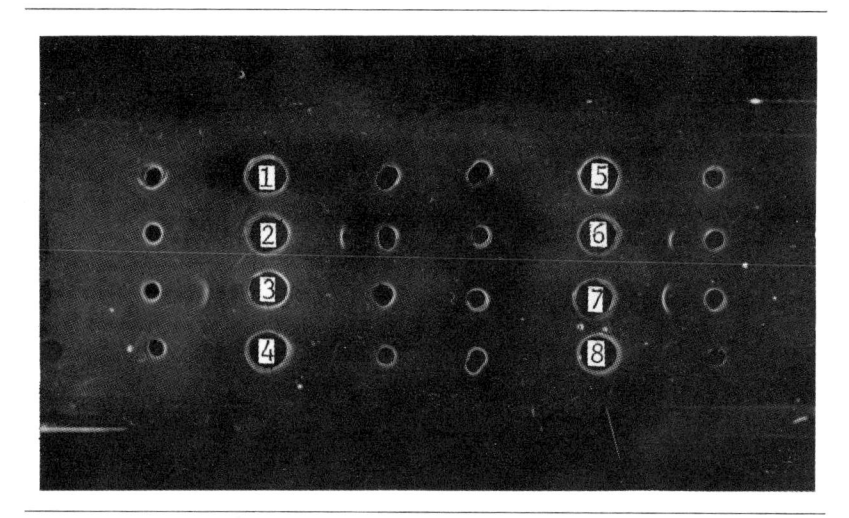

FIGURE 11: Two columns of test serum in the large wells with control antigen to the left and antibody to the right. Specimens 2, 4, 6, 7 and 8 have HB$_s$Ag whereas specimen 3 has anti-HB$_s$Ag.

b. *Advantages and disadvantages*

Counterelectrophoresis represents a modification of immunodiffusion with two advantages:

(1) Greater sensitivity because there is an increased concentration of reactants at the precipitation site. The antigen and antibody each move in a given direction in fairly narrow bands instead of diffusing in a radial fashion.

(2) Speed. The reactants are moved toward one another by their electrophoretic mobility rather than by diffusion.

All specimens positive for antigen or antibody by CEP should be confirmed for specificity. This may be done easily and economically by AGD or rheophoresis.

c. *Pitfalls*

It is difficult to differentiate a false positive from a true positive on CEP. The frequency of their occurrence depends on the specificity of the antiserum used. Most of the currently available commercial anti-HB$_s$Ag appear to have minimal reactants against nonspecific proteins.

Antibody from a single human donor or a pool of several human donors will occasionally show nonspecific precipitin lines. In our screening of sera of hospital patients using human source anti-HB$_s$Ag, we have identified 18 serum specimens which contain an antigen not identical with HB$_s$Ag. HB$_s$Ag inoculated into animals results in a much higher titered antibody response than usually occurs in human donors. This allows considerable dilution of the animal sera reducing the level of nonspecific reactants.

CEP kits should be used as complete systems. Reagents from different manufacturers should not be mixed or interchanged unless the formulations are known and found to be alike.[25] Buffers of the same pH may vary in the amounts and kinds of salts used. The pH and molarity of the buffer used determine the voltage or current required for the optimal separation of serum proteins in agarose. The agarose plates in the kits have a well pattern of calculated size, shape and distance between wells which should detect weak as well as strong antigens when tested against the antibody supplied. The reactants will form a precipitin line at the point where they meet at optimal relative concentrations. Minimally weak antigens will not form precipitin lines when the antibody exceeds the optimal relative concentration; likewise, a strong antigen will not form a precipitin line in the presence of a weak antibody. The sensitivity of a CEP system is often judged by how well it can detect weak antigens, but the possibility of missing strong antigens has been generally overlooked as being a problem. The fact that this does occur must be pointed out. We encountered one specimen recently in which the serum specimen detected by a commercially available kit was reported as negative but the same specimen was strongly positive in our system. In an effort to show how weak antibodies in closely approximated CEP wells may miss strong antigens, we varied the amount of HB$_s$Ag/anti-HB$_s$Ag ratio in the system in three ways:

(1) By making serum dilutions (Figure 12);

(2) By decreasing the size of the antigen well (Figure 13); and

(3) By increasing the distance between reactant wells (Figure 14).

All of these modifications that resulted in relative reduction of HB$_s$Ag allowed precipitation to take place.

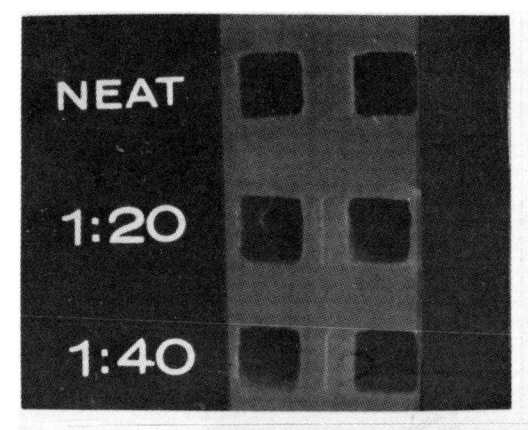

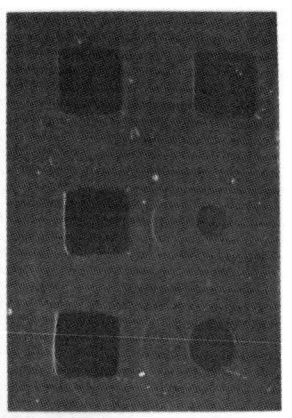

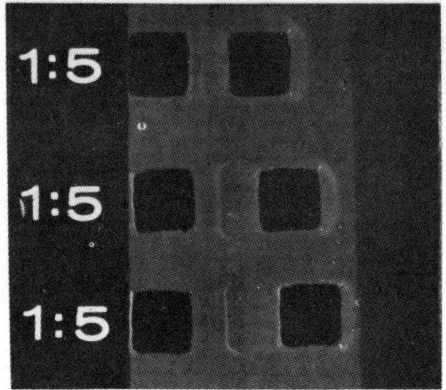

FIGURE 12: Pattern of commercial CEP plate showing negative reaction in top well with undilute test serum because of antigen excess. 1:20 and 1:40 dilutions, however, give obvious precipitation arcs.

FIGURE 13: The top well has undilute strongly positive serum which forms soluble complexes when the well size and distance provided in the kit are used (top). Smaller antigen wells give good precipitation arcs.

FIGURE 14: Using the well pattern and antibody of the commercial kit, a 1:5 dilution of the test serum gives a faint arc that is accentuated by spacing the wells further apart.

4. **Complement fixation (CF)**

   a. *Principle*

   Complement fixation is a time honored, sensitive method of detection of either antigen or antibody. The detection of one requires a known dilution of the other. The test is based on the principle that a combination of antigen and antibody will bind or "fix" complement. When there is no antigen to combine with the antibody, complement will remain free. Therefore, the presence or absence of free complement can be used to tell if an antigen-antibody complex has been formed.

The indicator system to test for free complement is sheep erythrocytes, to which is bound antibody to sheep erythrocytes. These cells are referred to as sensitized. The presence of free complement will cause the sensitized erythrocytes to lyse. When free complement is absent the cells will remain intact.

b. *Advantages and disadvantages*

Complement fixation is theoretically a great deal more sensitive than CEP or RHEO, but in practice with respect to detection of positive cases, CF is comparable in sensitivity to rheophoresis and CEP in testing for HB_sAg. The advantages are that it is quantitative and can be automated.[3,17] However, the antibody to be used must be of the complement-binding type, and antibody consumption is high in the test. Other disadvantages which have prevented this method from being widely used are:

(1) The test is time consuming.

(2) A prozone effect is encountered frequently.

(3) The sensitivity and reproducibility varies markedly from laboratory to laboratory.

5. **Hemagglutination inhibition (HAI)**

a. *Principle*

Purified HB_sAg is coated onto erythrocytes using chromium chloride as a coupling agent. The coated erythrocytes will agglutinate in the presence of a very small amount of carefully titered anti-HB_sAg. When test serum is incubated with the titered anti-HB_sAg, and the mixture is subsequently incubated with the coated cells, the antibody will be "neutralized" by any HB_sAg in the test serum, preventing it from agglutinating the coated cells.[3,28]

b. *Advantages and disadvantages*

The test is quantitative, specific, sensitive, simple to perform, and fairly rapid. The HAI method for detecting HB_sAg has been found to be very sensitive in the hands of investigators who are experienced in the technique. For routine testing purposes, the purified antigen used for coating the cells should be a pool of *ad* and *ay* particles while the antibody used should contain both anti-*ad* and anti-*ay*. Purified antigen and antigen coated cells are commercially available as serotype *ad, ay,* or as combinations of the two. Purified antigen is expensive. However, when calculated on a cost/test basis, it is less costly than CEP kits. The coated cells are very expensive but offer the advantage of being consistent in coating from lot to lot.

Test samples also may be examined for the presence of anti-HB_sAg by the direct agglutination of the HB_sAg coated cells or hemagglutination (HA). This is an extremely sensitive method for detecting anti-HB_sAg which has not been widely used, but has been very valuable in special studies.

c. *Pitfalls*

Successful reproducibility of test results is dependent upon consistency in the coating of cells from batch to batch. Consistency in coating of cells can be achieved if careful attention is given to factors which might interfere with the coating process;[3] i.e., fresh donor blood must be properly oxygenated, saline wash bottle must be free from bacterial growth, chromium chloride solution may be too old, etc. It has been reported that not all donors have coatable cells, therefore a single continual donor whose cells coat well would be advantageous.

6. **Reverse passive hemagglutination (RPHA)**

a. *Principle*

Reverse passive hemagglutination is a test system in which purified specific antibody is attached to fixed erythrocytes. The antibody-coated (or "reverse" coated) erythrocytes will agglutinate when exposed to sufficient specific antigen.[5,6] This very sensitive technique has been applied to HB_sAg.[15]

The procedure recently has been made available on a commercial basis and, although many laboratories participated in testing and evaluating the method prior to licensure, there have been a few modifications just before releases that we have not had the opportunity to test.

The technique utilizes microtiter plates[26] and requires 2 hours of settling time. The endpoint is ready by identifying the diffuse settling pattern of agglutinated erythrocytes. In earlier testing of the technique, we found that endpoint reading was easier in V-bottom plates and incubation time was only 20 minutes if the plates were centrifuged and set at an angle. The endpoint after centrifugation is determined by whether the erythrocytes stay in a button at the base or stream.[3]

b. *Advantages and disadvantages*

The hemagglutination technique is one of the more rapid procedures and its sensitivity approaches that of RIA. It lends itself well to quantitation, although at the present time the titer of HB_sAg may have no pracial importance.

On the disadvantage side, the method is quite costly, exceeding RIA in cost per test. A few false positive results may be encountered, but far less than one might anticipate. False positives can be excluded by a blocking technique in which one adds antibody supplied in a separate kit to the test serum, and titrates the mixture in parallel with the test serum to which has been added nonantibody control serum. Since the blocking kit is too expensive to utilize on every positive test in a hospital environment, it would be preferable to confirm positive results with rheophoresis, using the blocking test for those sera positive by hemagglutination but negative by RHEO. All sera giving a positive hemagglutination result should have confirmatory testing or be referred to as "presumptive positive."

c. *Pitfalls*

The microtiter dilutors in hemagglutination are calibrated to transfer liquid assuming no contact with the side of the microtiter well by the dilutors. Brushing the dilutor against the well will cause error in titer of HB_sAg.

The settling of the erythrocytes should take place in a vibration-free area. Continual vibration, shaking, or jarring may make positive sera appear negative.

The kit provides no cell control. Theoretically, a serum may have an erythrocyte antibody although we have never encountered one. The practice of confirmation of positive results eliminates this problem.

II. Hepatitis B (Core) Antigen and Antibody

The principle thrust of hepatitis B testing has been toward identification of what seems to be excess coat material of the virus (surface antigen). The life cycle of the hepatitis virus and the relationship of the virus to the surface antigen is unclear, but the larger "Dane" particle would appear to be a more likely candidate for the virus[7] while the HB_sAg particle seems to be an excess of the same material that coats the Dane particle.[1] The liver cell nucleus appears to be the site of origin of the virus,[8, 13] whereas the cytoplasm is the principle area where HB_sAg can be demonstrated.[9, 10, 27] Recently, there has been a demonstration of antibody to the core of the Dane particle developing in patients with acute viral hepatitis. Although detection of this antibody in rising titer would appear to have tremendous clinical importance, practical application of the test must await a method of harvesting core particles of the hepatitis-B virus.

In summary, hepatitis antigen testing has become a common laboratory procedure, but often the procedure is performed in a cookbook fashion that overlooks certain pitfalls and ignores the necessity of confirmatory testing. In our laboratory all sera to be tested are concentrated 10-fold with polyacrilamide gel and screened by counterelectrophoresis. All positive results are confirmed by rheophoresis. All negative sera are tested by RIA and those found to be positive are retested by blocking for confirmation. A laboratory that has fewer positive specimens than we do might more profitably test only by hemagglutination, confirming positive results with RHEO or blocking techniques. We would expect that tests more specifically directed toward identification of antibody response to the actual virus ultimately will be available and of greater value to blood donor facilities.

REFERENCES

1. Almeida JD: New antigen-antibody system in Australia-antigen-positive hepatitis. *Lancet* **2**:1225-1227,1971b.
2. Ashcavai M, Peters RL: Hepatitis-associated antigen: Improved sensitivity in detection. *Am. J. Clin. Path.* **55**(3):262-268, 1971.
3. Ashcavai M, Peters RL: Manual for Hepatitis B Antigen Testing. W. B. Saunders Co. 1973.
4. Blumberg BS, Gerstley BJS, Hungerford DA, et al: A serum antigen (Australia antigen) in Down's syndrome, leukemia, and hepatitis. *Ann. Int. Med.* **66**:924-931, 1967.
5. Cook RJ: Reversed passive hemagglutination systems for the estimation of tetanus toxins and antitoxins. *Immunology* **8**:74, 1965.
6. Cook RJ: Titration of *Clostridium oedematiens* antitoxin by reversed passive hemagglutination. *Immunology* **9**:249, 1965.
7. Dane DS, Cameron CH, Briggs M: Virus-like particles in serum of patients with Australia-antigen-associated hepatitis. *Lancet* **1**:695, 1970.

8. Dunn AEG, Peters RL, Schweitzer IL: An ultrastructural study of liver explants from infants with vertically transmitted hepatitis. *Exp. Mol. Path.* **19**(1):113-126, 1973.
9. Edgington TS, Ritt DJ: Intrahepatic expression of serum hepatitis virus-associated antigens. *J. Exp. Med.* **134**:871-885 (Oct. 1) 1971.
10. Gerber MA, Schaffner F, Paronetto F: Immune-electron microscopy of hepatitis B antigen in liver. *Proc. Soc. Exp. Biol. Med.* **140**:1334-1339, 1972.
11. Hirata AA, Brandriss MW: Passive hemagglutination procedures for protein and polysaccharide antigens using erythrocytes stabilized by aldehydes. *J. Immunonogy* **100**:64, 1968.
12. Hoofnagle JH, Gerety RJ, Barker LF: Antibody to hepatitis-B-virus core in man. *Lancet* **2**:869-873, 1973.
13. Huang SN: Hepatitis-associated antigen hepatitis: an electron microscopic study of virus-like particles in liver cells *Am. J. Path.* **64**:483-491, 1971.
14. Jambazian A, Holper JC: Rheophoresis: A sensitive immunodiffusion method for detection of hepatitis-associated antigen. *Proc. Soc. Exp. Biol. & Med.* **140**:560-564, 1972.
15. Juji T, Yokochi T: Hemagglutination technique and erythrocyte coated with specific antibody for detection of Australia antigen. *Japan J. Exp. Med.* **39**:615-620, 1969.
16. Kissling RE, Barker L: Evaluation of assay methods for hepatitis associated antigen. *Applied Microbiology* **23**(6):1037-1046, 1972.
17. Kwak KS, Gitnick GL, Sturgeon P: Hepatitis-associated antigen screening by automated complement fixation: comparison with manual methods. *Am. J. Clin. Path.* **59**:41-48, 1973.
18. LeBouvier GL: The heterogeneity of Australia antigen. *J. Inf. Dis.* **123**(6): 671-675, 1971.
19. Mazzur S, Falker D, Blumberg BS: Geographical variation of the "w" subtype of Australia antigen. *Nature New Biol.* **243**:44-47, 1973.
20. Mosley JW, Edwards VM, Wapplehorst B, et al: Hepatitis B virus subtypes *ad* and *ay* among blood donors in the greater Los Angeles area. In press. *Transfusion* July-Aug, 1974.
21. Prince AM: An antigen detected in blood during the incubation period of serum hepatitis. *Proc. Nat. Acad. Sci.* **60**:814-821, 1968.
22. Prince AM, Burke K: Serum hepatitis antigen (SH): Rapid detection by high voltage immunoelectroosmophosresis. *Science* **169**: 593-595, 1970.

23. Roche JK, Stengle JM: Comparison of the sensitivities of the newer detection systems for hepatitis B antigen. *Transfusion* **13**(5): 258-265, 1973.
24. Schmidt NJ, Lennette EH: Complement fixation and immunodiffusion tests for assay of hepatitis-associated "Australia" antigen and antibodies. *J. Immunol.* **105**(3):604-613, 1970.
25. Schmidt NJ, Lennette EH: Evaluation of various antisera and gels for detection of hepatitis-associated antigen by immunodiffusion and immunoelectroosmophoresis. *Am. J. Clin. Path.* **58**(3):317-325, 1972.
26. Sever JL: Application of microtechnique to viral serological investigations. *J. Immunology* **88**:320, 1962.
27. Stein O, Fainaru M, Stein Y: Visualization of virus-like particles in endoplasmic reticulum of hepatocytes of Australia antigen carriers. *Lab. Invest.* **26**:262-269, 1972.
28. Vyas GN, Mason MA, Williams EW: Detection of hepatitis B antigen and antibodies by hemagglutination assay. *Hepatitis and Blood Transfusion.* Vyas GN, Perkins HA, Schmidt R, (eds.) *Grune and Stratton, 1972.*

MICROEMBOLIZATION AND BLOOD TRANSFUSION
R. Thomas Solis

PARTICULATE microembolization has been known to occur during transfusion of stored blood since the beginning of blood banking.[9, 20] As a result, a wide variety of blood filters consisting of reusable wire mesh, gauze and other materials were used to remove the amorphous material which develops in stored blood.[8] By the mid 1950's the currently used disposable plastic clot mesh filters with a pore size of 170 μ were in wide spread use.[51] Although considerable particulate material smaller than the pore size was known to pass through these filters,[26] they were preferred because of the rapid flow rates with which they allow stored blood to be infused.[52]

The clinical significance of the particulate material which remained in stored blood after passage through the clot mesh filters was not apparent until 1961, when Swank introduced the screen filtration pressure (SFP) technique to quantitate the microaggregates in stored blood.[45] He noted that the SFP, which is the pressure required to force blood through a 20 μ pore mesh filter,[49] increased during the first 2 to 10 days of storage of blood in ACD under blood bank conditions. He demonstrated microscopically that the SFP increased in association with the aggregation of leukocytes and platelets. The SFP remained high after passage through clot mesh filters but was reduced to normal levels after passage through filters consisting of glass, Nylon and Dacron wool.

In subsequent clinical studies, the high SFP in stored blood used to prime blood oxygenators prior to cardiopulmonary bypass was noted to fall to normal after passage through the patient.[48] In addition, the SFP of blood drawn from patients receiving massive blood transfusions was shown to fall progressively from central venous to arterial to peripheral venous samples[28]. These studies implied that the particulate material which the SFP method detects was removed by the microcirculation of the recipient and are consistent with the histologic finding of multiple pulmonary microemboli in patients who receive massive blood transfusions.[7, 17, 31, 36]

Clinical studies of combat casualties have demonstrated a significant arterial hypoxemia in patients receiving over 8 units of stored blood.[28, 40] These have implicated the microaggregates in stored blood in the development of pulmonary insufficiency after trauma. However, many complicating factors are usually associated with massive transfusion in man which may also contribute to the development of pulmonary insufficiency.[44] These include shock, fat embolism, overhydration, and pulmonary trauma per se. As a result, most of the evidence suggesting that infusion of the microaggregates in stored blood may be harmful to the recipient has been based on experimental studies of laboratory animals.

Transfusion of stored blood with a high SFP causes pulmonary hypertension[1, 16, 30] and transient increases in dead space ventilation[47] in dogs and alterations in the electroencephalogram of cats.[15] Ultrastructural studies of the lungs of dogs receiving large quantities of stored blood filtered with the standard clot filter have shown lesions similar to those noted after hemorrhagic shock.[6] These pulmonary lesions,[6] which consist of interstitial edema, degeneration of the capillary endothelial and type I alveolar cells, and evidence of obstruction of pulmonary blood flow[1, 30] can be prevented by effective filtration of the stored blood.

Although much information has been obtained with canine models, primate studies are of greater interest because the microaggregates which develop in baboon blood during storage are similar to those of man, while those in canine blood are smaller.[22] Transfusion of stored autologous baboon blood into an isolated lung perfused *in situ* has been found to increase the pulmonary vascular resistance and lung water and to decrease arterial oxygenation.[4] On the other hand, massive exchange transfusion with stored type-specific blood in unanesthetized baboons after a two-hour period of severe hypotension did not cause alterations in arterial blood oxygenation within one hour.[22] These studies demonstrate that transfusion of stored blood causes alterations in primate pulmonary function and that the unanesthetized baboon can compensate for these effects immediately after the transfusion. The chronic effects of massive transfusion on the intact baboon are under study; similarly, the effects of the newer blood filters in preventing the development of the abnormalities in the isolated lung model are currently under investigation.

It is well established that microembolization occurs as a result of blood transfusions; however, quantitation of these particles has been limited because of their wide size range and marked instability. The SFP method is sensitive to adhesiveness as well as to aggregation of blood cells and platelets and does not indicate the quantity of material which obstructs the 20 μ pore filter.[49] Another method of quantitation of the particulate material consists of weighing the amount of material retained by a filter.[26, 28, 31, 37] In studies of combat casualties receiving blood transfusions, Moseley and Doty found that as much as 5 g of material was retained by the standard blood transfusion filter (170 μ pore mesh) during filtration of a unit of blood.[31] However, this method does not reflect the smaller particles which pass through the filters, nor the labile particles larger than the pore size of the filter which break up and pass through mesh filters. Many turbidimetric,[5, 33] filtration,[24] and other techniques[12, 39] have been developed for the study of platelet aggregation, but these methods are restricted to the study of aggregates in plasma and do not give quantitative information on the size and number of aggregates in blood.

In order to quantitate particulate material in blood, we have used an electronic particle size analyzer to measure the size and number of microaggregates in blood. The operation of the instrument and analysis of data are described in detail elsewhere.[41, 44] Briefly, the instrument simultaneously counts the number of particles in 15 pre-set channels, each of which detects particles twice the size of the previous channel. As a result, an analysis can be obtained over a wide size range immediately after dilution of a sample of blood or plasma in a diluent.

The size distribution data may be presented either as the number or the volume of particles detected in each channel or as the cumulative number or volume of particles detected within a given size range. The volume of particles, which is calculated by multiplying the number counted by the mean size in μ^3 of particles detected in a given channel of the instrument, has been found to be the most convenient means of presenting and analyzing the data.[44] This is because it allows calculation of the cumulative mass of particles detected over a wide size range. This is illustrated in Figure 1 where the differential volume size distribution of platelets in platelet-rich plasma (PRP) with and without aggregation induced by adenosine diphosphate (ADP) is plotted. Although the modal size of the platelets increased from 2.5 to 64 μ as a result of aggregation, the cumulative volume of aggregates which were formed in the ADP-treated plasma (i.e. particles larger than 13 μ) did not differ from that of the platelets which aggregated. This demonstrates that electronic size measurements can be made of platelet aggregates in plasma. However, electronic measurements of microaggregates larger than leukocytes in non-hemolyzed suspensions of blood are limited to particles larger than 32 μ because of the marked gain in secondary coincidence counts due to erythrocytes in the channels measuring particles 13 to 25 μ in size.[44]

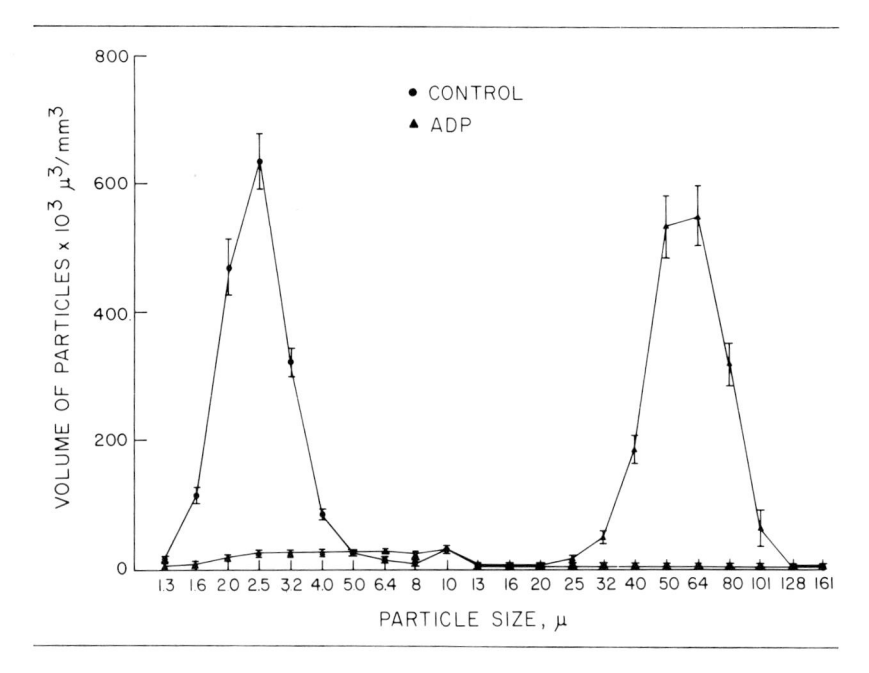

FIGURE 1: Differential volume size distribution of platelets and platelet aggregates in platelet-rich plasma (PRP). Buffered saline with and without (control) ADP (2 × 10⁻⁶M) was added to aliquots of PRP (1:9 by volume), which were then shaken for 60 seconds prior to dilution in Isoton for analysis. Particles smaller than 13 μ were measured with a 70 μ aperture (1:6,000 dilution); particles 13 μ and larger were measured with a 400 μ aperture (1:200 dilution). Although the cumulative number of particles was reduced from 198 × 10³ to 14 × 10³/mm³ as a result of aggregation, the cumulative volume of aggregates formed did not differ from that of the non-aggregated platelets which disappeared. (mean ± S.E., n=8).

In order to reduce the lower limit of the size measurements of microaggregates in blood to 13 μ, we have added saponin[41] or Zap-Isoton[43] (Coulter Electronics, Hialeah, Fla.) to the diluent to lyse erythrocytes. Although saponin accelerates the dissociation of larger platelet aggregates after dilution in saline and prevents the accumulation of smaller aggregates, the measurements made immediately after dilution in saline containing saponin are not significantly different from control measurements (Figure 2). As a result, electronic measurements can be made of platelet aggregates 13 μ and larger in blood immediately following lysis of erythrocytes by saponin in the diluent but before significant dissociation of aggregates has occurred (Figure 3).

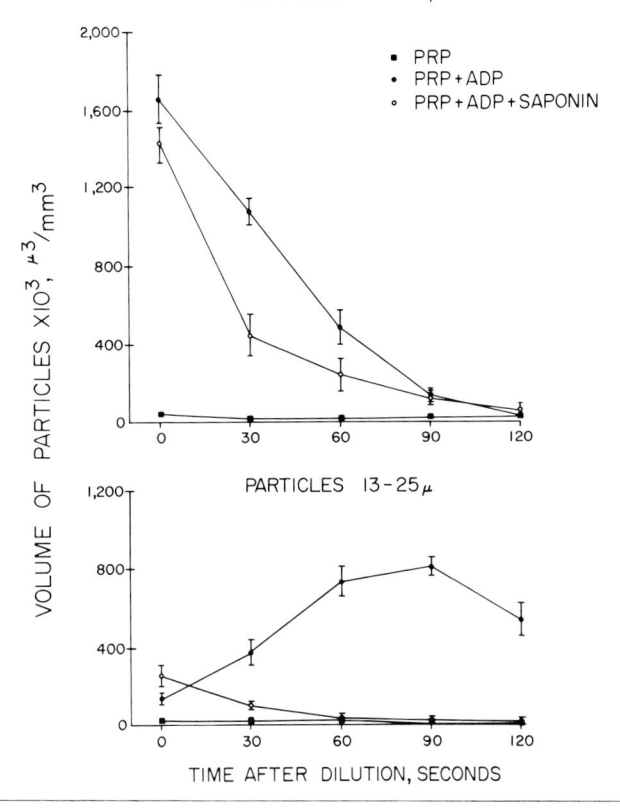

FIGURE 2: Effect of saponin on deaggregation of platelets in plasma following dilution in isotonic saline. The cumulative volume of particles 32 to 80 μ (top panel) and 13 to 25 μ in size (bottom panel) was measured immediately (time 0), and every 30 seconds for two minutes, after dilution of control PRP in saline (PRP) or PRP containing ADP-(2×10^{-6}M)-induced platelet aggregates in saline (PRP + ADP) or in saline containing saponin (500 mg/L) (PRP + ADP + Saponin) (mean ± S.E., n=8).

The physical characteristics of the microaggregates in stored blood differ markedly from those of platelet aggregates which can be induced in fresh blood by ADP. This is shown in Figure 4 where the dissociation of microaggregates in a unit of stored blood after dilution in saline containing increasing concentrations of saponin is compared to that of platelet aggregates induced in fresh blood by ADP. As noted in Figure 2 with the platelet aggregates induced in plasma, saponin, which is a strong surface active agent,[25] increased the dissociation of the

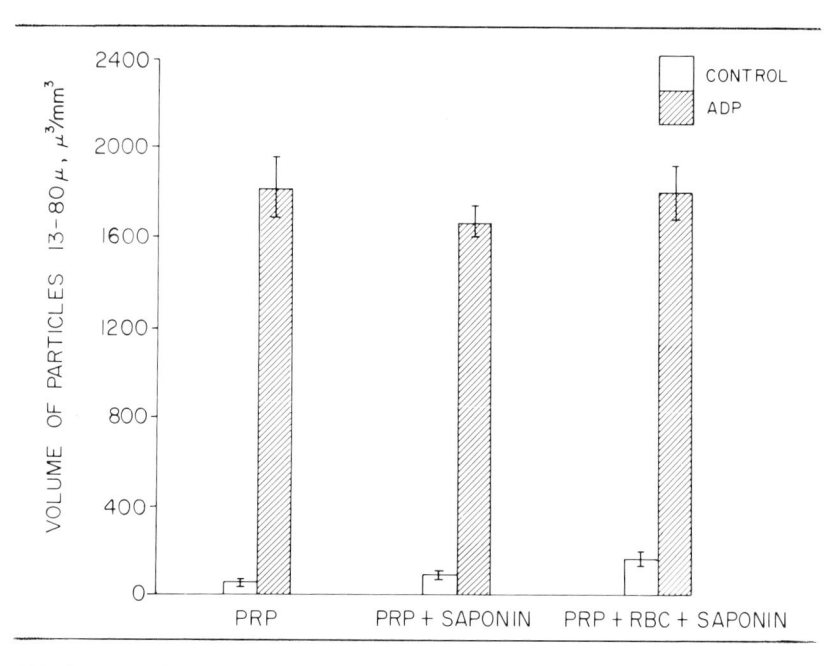

FIGURE 3: Effect of hemolysis of erythrocytes after dilution in saline containing saponin on electronic measurements of platelet aggregates. In order to assure that the platelet concentration and reactivity in PRP and in blood were comparable, autologous platelet-poor plasma or saline-washed erythrocytes were added to platelet-rich plasma prior to induction of platelet aggregation by ADP as shown in Figure 1. The data show that the cumulative volume of platelet aggregates measured immediately following dilution of PRP in saline without saponin (PRP) was not different from that measured following dilution of PRP in saline containing saponin (500 mg/L)(PRP + Saponin) nor from that measured following dilution of PRP containing saline-washed red cells (hematocrit = 38%) in the saline-saponin diluent (PRP + RBC + Saponin).

platelet aggregates in blood. In contrast, the microaggregates in the stored blood remained relatively stable as the saponin concentration was increased. In other studies of these two types of microaggregates after exposure to ethylenediaminetetracetate[43] or to alterations in pH,[44] the microaggregates in the stored blood were noted to be more resistant to dissociation *in vitro*. This indicates that the microaggregates which develop in stored blood are more tightly bound than are acutely induced platelet aggregates and would presumably be more resistant to dissociation *in vivo*.

Electronic measurements of blood during storage under blood bank conditions demonstrate that there is a progressive increase in the cumu-

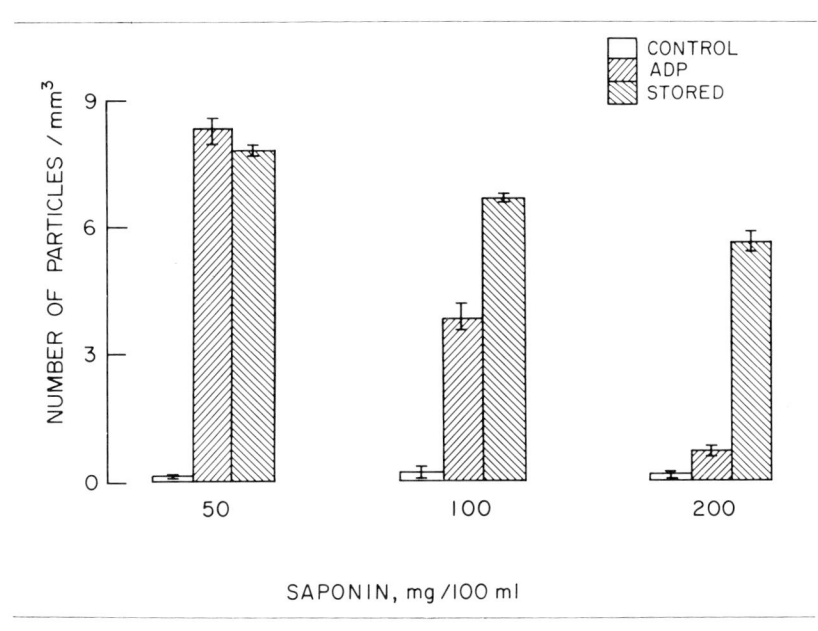

FIGURE 4: Effect of increasing the saponin concentration in the saline diluent on the cumulative number of particles 32-80 μ in size measured 30 seconds after dilution of (1) stored blood (Stored), (2) fresh sodium-citrated (0.32%) human blood 60 seconds after adding ADP in buffered saline (2×10^{-6}M) (ADP), and (3) fresh citrated blood (Control) 1 min. after adding an equal volume of saline without ADP to blood (1:10).(mean ± S.E., n=8).

lative volume of microaggregates during the 21-day storage period in ACD (Figure 5). Coincident with the development of the microaggregates shown in Figure 5, there was a progressive reduction in absolute granulocyte count obtained by hemocytometry and differential staining, while the lymphocyte count remained unchanged.[44] The hemocytometry platelet counts fell only during the first week of storage. In other studies, the electronic measurements demonstrated that the reduction in the cumulative volume of particles in the size range of leukocytes (5-10 μ in equivalent spherical diameter) during storage was approximately equal to that of the microaggregates which developed (Figure 6). Since the measurements shown in Figures 5 and 6 were made two minutes after dilution in saline containing saponin, they represent the volume of particles that are most resistant to deaggregation and would presumably be most damaging to the tissue to which they embolize.

These electronic measurements confirm earlier studies using light

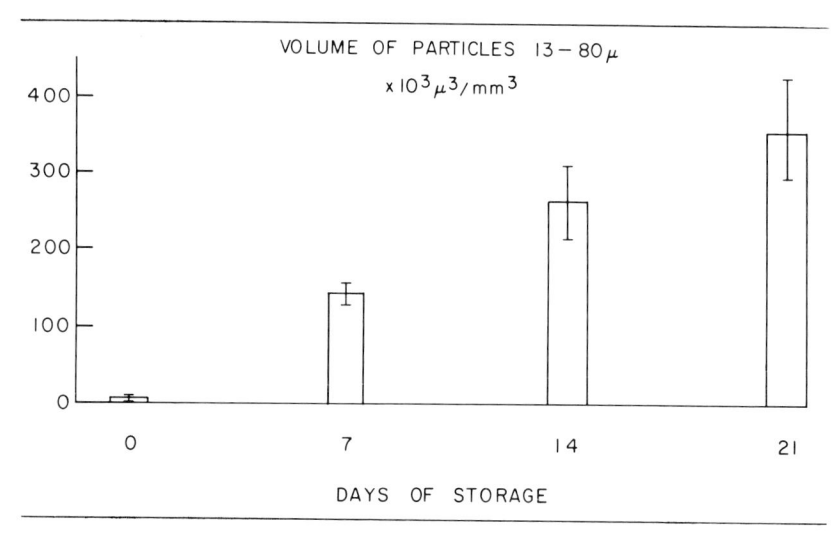

FIGURE 5: Development of microaggregates during storage. Changes in cumulative volume of microaggregates 13 to 80 μ in size in eight units of blood drawn into ACD are plotted against the days of storage at 4-6 C. The measurements were made 2 minutes after dilution in saline containing saponin (200 mg/100 ml).

microscopy and special staining techniques which demonstrated that platelets and leukocytes aggregate during storage of blood under blood bank conditions.[9, 18, 21, 45, 50] Lymphocytes are relatively non-adhesive[10] and remain functional during most of the 21 days of storage in ACD.[27] In contrast, platelets and granulocytes rapidly lose their viability during storage and become adhesive.[2, 21, 50] As a result of their adhesiveness, these components stick to each other when they settle into the buffy coat.[45] Ultrastructural studies demonstrate that during the first few days of storage only platelet aggregates are noted, while subsequently, the granulocytes begin to degenerate and lose their cell membranes.[53] The resulting microaggregates are complex particles which consist of platelets and the nuclear material of granulocyte but not of fibrin and lymphocytes.[53]

Since the microaggregates consist of platelets and leukocytes, the extent of formation of these particles during storage of various blood components is dependent on their initial concentration prior to storage.[45] This is shown in Figure 7 where the cumulative volume of microaggregates which developed in various blood components prepared by differential centrifugation is plotted against the change in hemocytometry platelet and leukocyte counts in the components during the storage period. These studies indicate that removal of platelets and

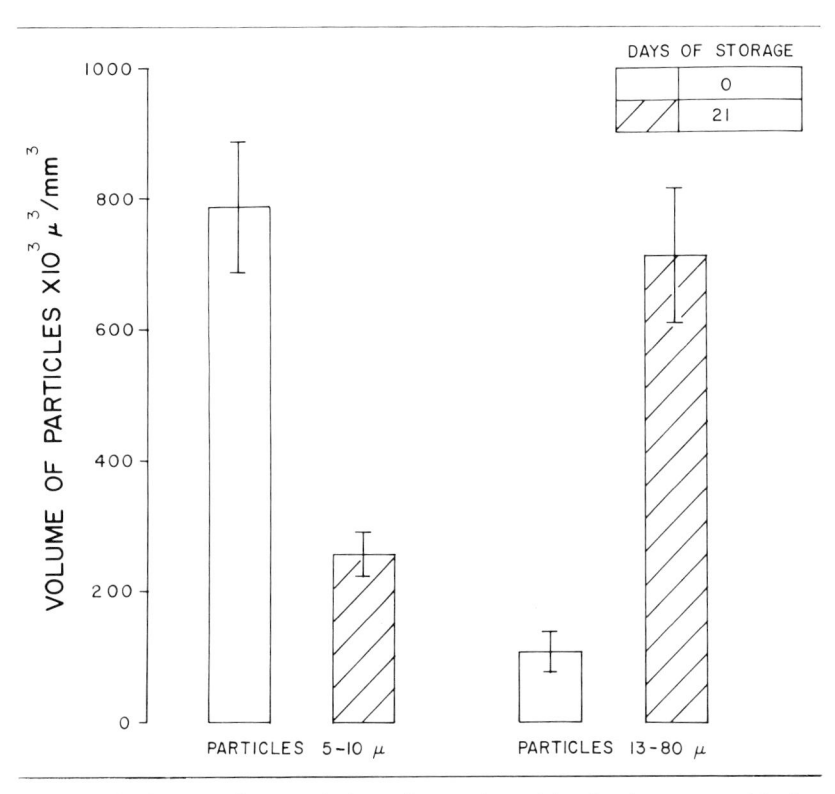

FIGURE 6: Changes in cumulative volume of particles in size range of leukocytes (particles 5-10 μ) and of microaggregates (particles 13-80 μ) during storage of six units of human bloood in ACD plastic bags at 4-6 C for 21 days. (mean ± S.E.).

granulocytes for other purposes prior to storage will indirectly reduce the extent of microembolization which would occur when the unit is subsequently transfused. However, many other factors affect microaggregate formation. Blood drawn into heparin or CPD anti-coagulant develops more platelet aggregates than with ACD early in storage,[44, 48] while pretreatment of blood with prostaglandin E_1 reduces the formation of aggregates and improves the recovery of platelets in plasma.[3, 38] In addition, the technique with which the blood was drawn, the medical and drug history of the donor, and the conditions of storage are probably important factors in microaggregate formation.[19, 37]

Since the microaggregates have a density similar to that of platelets and leukocytes, they settle into the buffy coat after a hard centrifugation.[45] Removal of the buffy coat after such centrifugation renders the

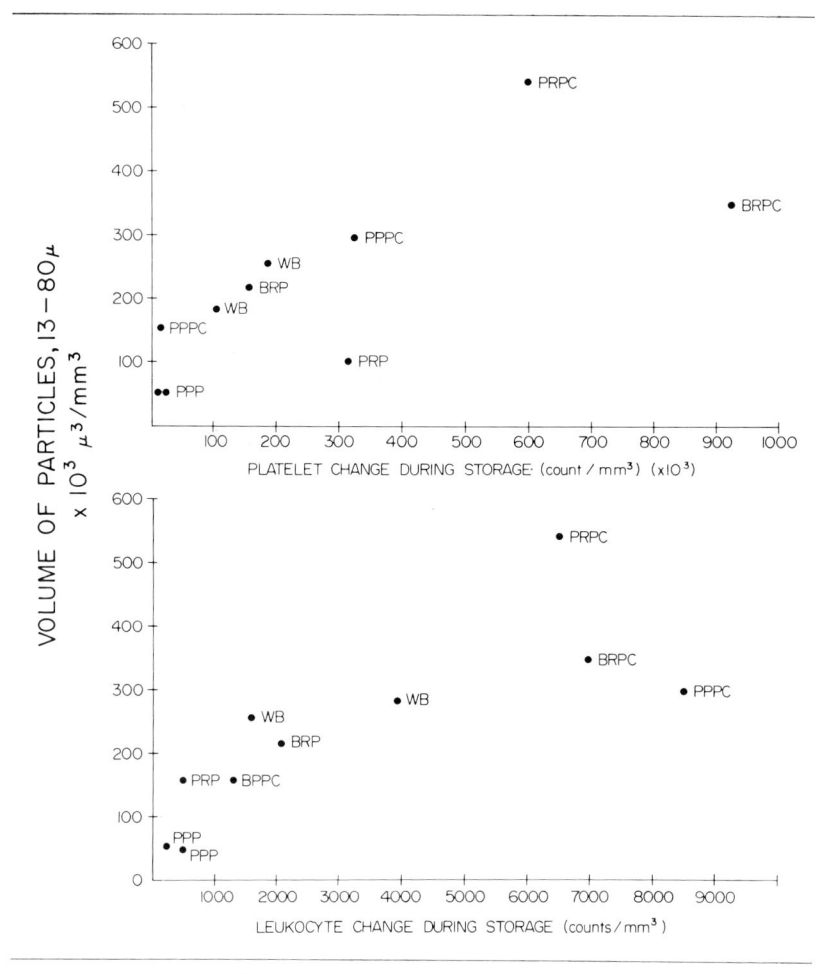

FIGURE 7: Microaggregate formation in various blood components. Cumulative volume of microaggregates measured 21 days after storage at 4-6 C plotted against reductions in hemocytometry platelet (top panel) and leukocyte (bottom panel) counts. The components were prepared by differential centrifugation after drawing 16 units of human blood into ACD anticoagulant. (PPP = platelet-poor plasma; PRP = platelet-rich plasma; BRP = platelet and buffy-coat rich plasma; PPPC = platelet-poor packed cells; PRPC = platelet-rich packed cells; BRPC = buffy-coat rich packed cells; WB = whole blood). Each point represents the mean of measurements of eight separate components.

resuspended red cells and plasma relatively free of microaggregates (Figure 8). Because of their adhesiveness, the microaggregates smaller than 80 μ, which would ordinarily pass through the standard clot filter,

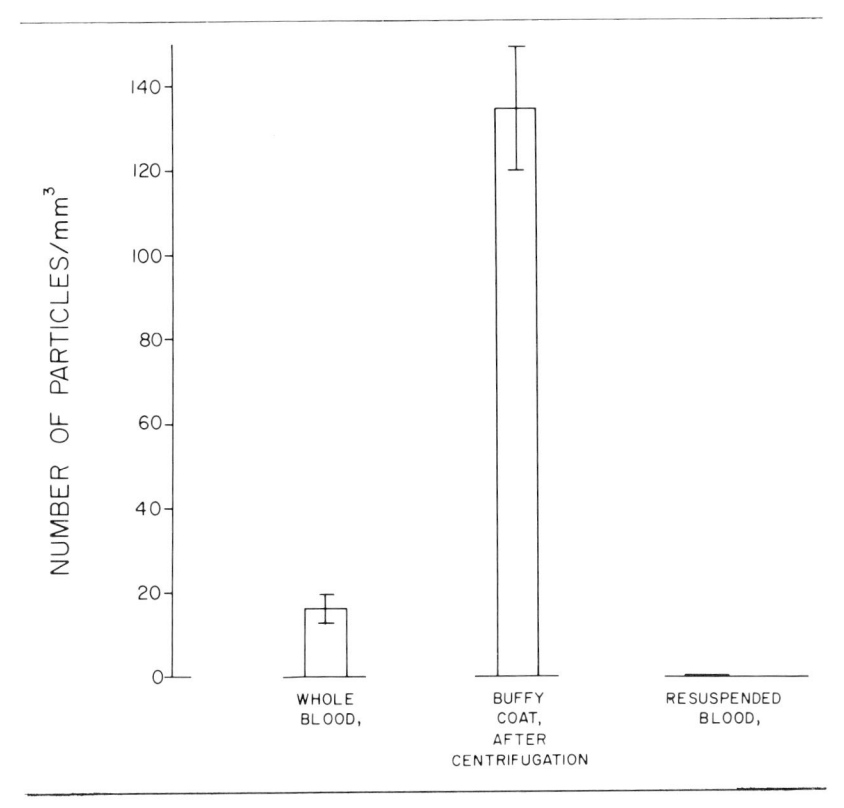

FIGURE 8: Effect of buffy-coat removal on microaggregate concentration in stored blood. Cumulative number of particles 32-80 μ in size in a unit of ACD human blood stored 21 days at 4-6 C; in buffy-coat after centrifugation (2,000 × g for 5 minutes), and in the resuspended plasma and red cells.

aggregate to form larger particles when they settle into the buffy coat during centrifugation.[44] As a result, centrifugation and resuspension of stored blood prior to filtration markedly increases the amount of particulate material which can be removed by the 170 μ pore mesh filter.[41] Another means of removing the microaggregates is to wash the blood. Quantitative studies have shown that either manual or automated methods of washing can remove up to 90%, by volume, of microaggregates from stored blood.[11]

Although many *in vitro* techniques can be used to remove or to prevent the formation of microaggregates, the simplest means of removal is by filtration. Previous studies with the electronic particle size analyzer have confirmed the early finding of Swank[45] that the standard clot mesh

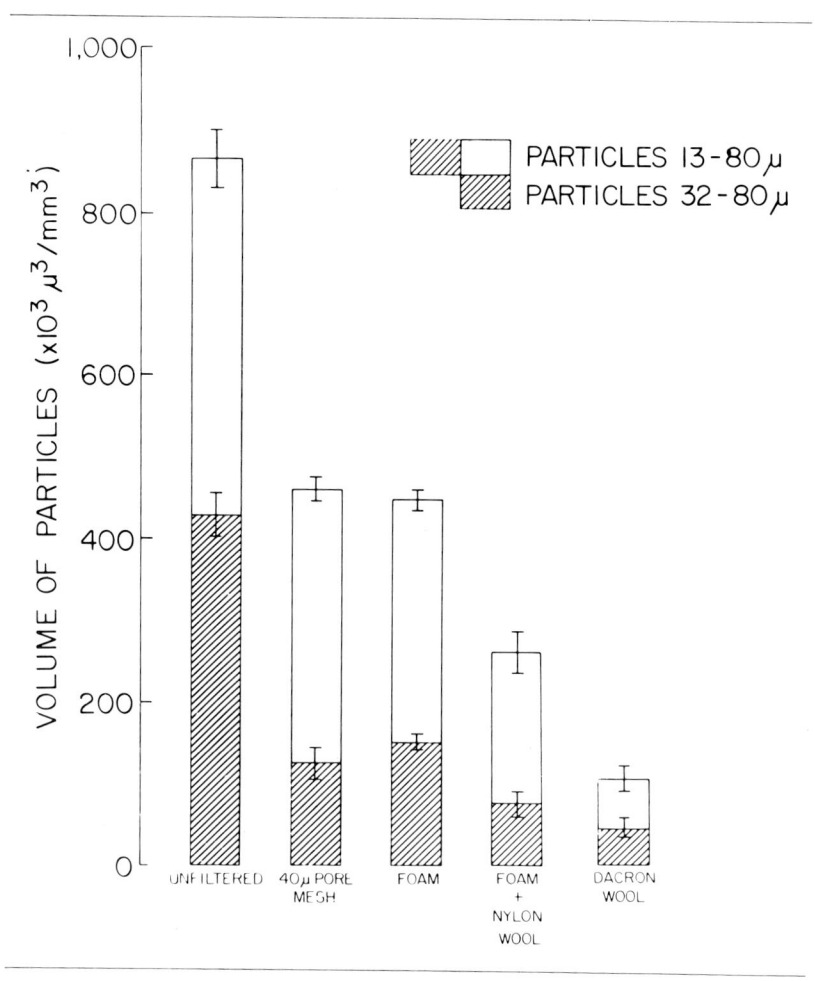

FIGURE 9: Filtration of microaggregates in stored blood. Cumulative volume of particles 13 to 80 and 32 to 80 μ in size in a large pool of type-specific outdated stored blood before and after passage through various blood transfusion filters. (40 μ pore mesh = Ultipore, Pall Corporation, Glen Cove, N. Y.; Foam = polyurethane foam filter, PF127, Bentley Laboratories, Santa Ana, Ca.; Foam + Nylon wool = The Microaggregate Blood Filter, Fenwal Laboratories, Morton Grove, Ill.; Dacron wool = Swank Transfusion Filter, Extracorporeal Medical Specialists; King of Prussia, Pa.)

filter with 170 μ pores cannot remove particles 80 μ and smaller from stored blood.[41] As a result of the clinical and experimental studies which indicated that the microaggregates may be harmful to the recipient,[1, 4, 6, 7, 14-17, 29, 31, 32, 46] a wide variety of blood filters are now

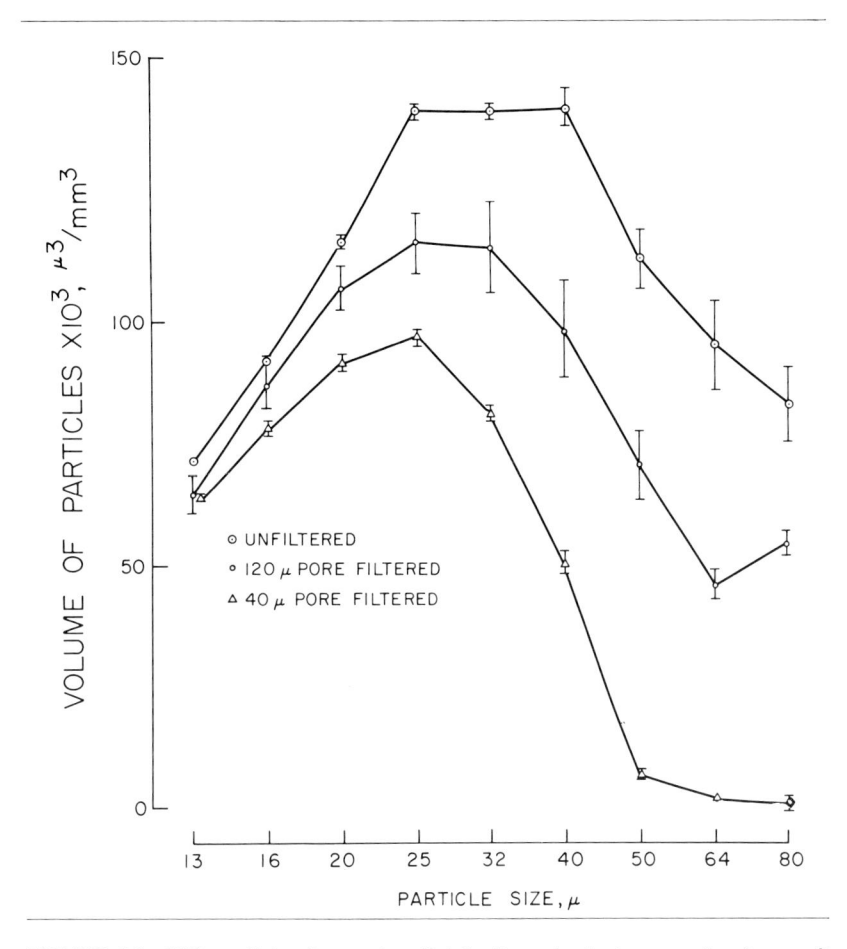

FIGURE 10: Differential volume size distribution of microaggregates in a unit of human blood stored 21 days in ACD at 4-6 C before and after passage through mesh filters with 120 and 40 μ pores.

commercially available which are more effective than the standard clot mesh filter.[28, 35, 41, 43] Figure 9 shows size distribution measurements of microaggregates in a large pool of outdated stored blood before and after passage through some of these newer blood filters. The 40 μ pore mesh filter,[35] was effective at removal of particles only 32 μ and larger. The size distribution of the microaggregates remaining after passage through the foam filter, which consists of three layers of polyurethane foam with decreasing pore sizes (150, 70 and 30 μ) was similar to that after passage through the 40 μ pore mesh filter. The foam-Nylon wool filter consists of a single layer of polyurethane foam with 150 μ pores and a layer of packed Nylon wool. It was more effective at removal of the smaller microaggregates than the 40 μ pore mesh and foam filter, but was less efficient than the Dacron wool filter.

The mechanism of filtration of these blood filters differs. Dacron wool functions by providing a large surface to which particles may stick. It is a "depth filter," and its efficiency is determined by the adhesiveness rather than the size of the particle being filtered. Thus the relatively non-adhesive platelets and leukocytes in fresh ACD blood are not removed, whereas those in heparinized blood, which are more adhesive, are removed by Dacron wool filtration.[1] In contrast, the 40 μ pore filter functions as a "surface filter" whose efficiency at particle removal is determined by the relation between the size of the pores and the size of the particles being filtered (Figure 10). The particle size measurements suggest that the foam filter functions as a surface filter whose efficiency is determined by the size of the smallest pore in the filtering elements. The foam-Nylon wool filter is a combination of a surface and depth filter; however, it is less efficient at particle removal than the Dacron wool filter.

Clinical experience with these more effective blood filters has been limited primarily to use during cardiopulmonary bypass.[14, 34, 35] However, Ruel et al studied traumatized patients receiving over 10 units of stored blood.[36] They noted a higher incidence of pulmonary insufficiency in patients who received blood administered through standard clot mesh filters than in patients whose blood had been administered though the 40 μ pore mesh filter. Lung biopsies obtained from patients whose blood was effectively filtered revealed no alterations,[7, 36] while those obtained from patients whose blood was filtered by the clot mesh filters had lesions similar to those noted previously in experimental animals.[6] Although these studies suggest that the microaggregates in stored blood may be damaging to the recipient, the clinical situations which require their effective removal remain to be determined. The lung has an enormous filtering capacity[13] and many patients have received large quantities of blood without pulmonary complications. The newer blood filters add to expense of medical care and are often difficult to use because of their tendency to develop an increased resistance to flow after filtration of one or two units.[42] However, in situations such as cardiopulmonary bypass, where infused microemboli would enter the systemic circulation prior to filtration by the lungs, and in transfusion of critically ill patients whose pulmonary reserve may be limited, the most effective filter should probably be used.

ACKNOWLEDGEMENT: This work was partially supported by U. S. Army Medical Research and Development Command contract #DADA 17-73-C-3149 and U. S. Public Health Service Grant (HL-138-37-03).

REFERENCES

1. Ashmore PG, Swank RL, Gallery R, et al: Effect of Dacron wool filtration on the microembolic phenomenon in extracorporeal circulation. *J. Thorac. Cardiovasc. Surg.* **63**:240, 1972.

2. Baldini M, Costea N, Dameshek W: The viability of stored human platelets. *Blood* **16**:1669, 1960.

3. Becker GA, Chalos MK, Tuccelli M, et al: Prostaglandin E_1 in preparation and storage of platelet concentrates. *Science* **175**:538, 1972.

4. Bennett SR, Geelhoed G, Hoye R, et al: Pulmonary injury resulting from perfusion with stored blood bank. *J. Surg. Res.* **13**:295, 1972.

5. Born GV: Quantitative investigations into the aggregation of blood platelets. *J. Physiol.* **162**:67P, 1962.

6. Connell RS, Swank RL: Pulmonary fine structure after hemorrhagic shock and transfusion of aging blood. In Jorn Ditzek and D. H. Lewis (Eds.): *Microcirculatory Approaches to Current Therapeutic Problems. Lung in Shock. Organ Transplantation. Diabetic Microangiopathy.* Symposia held simultaneously at the 6th European Conference on Microcirculation, Aalborg 1970. Basel: S. Karger, 1971, pp. 40-58.

7. Connell RS, Page US, Bartley TD, et al: The effect of Dacron wool filtration during cardiopulmonary bypass. *Ann. Thorac. Surg.* **15**:217, 1973.

8. DeGowin EL: Transfusion equipment. In DeGowin EL, Hardin RC, Alsever JB (Eds.): *Blood Transfusion.* Philadelphia: W. B. Saunders Co., 1949, pp. 515-539.

9. Fantus B: Therapy of Cook County Hospital; blood preservation technic. *J.A.M.A.* **111**:317, 1938.

10. Garvin JA: Factors affecting the adhesiveness of human leukocytes and platelets *in vitro*. *J. Exp. Med.* **114**:51, 1961.

11. Goldfinger D, Solis RT, Meryman HT: Microaggregates in frozen and saline washed red blood cells. *Transfusion.* In press, 1973.

12. Glynn MF, Movat HZ, Murphy EA, et al: Study of platelet adhesiveness and aggregation, with latex particles. *J. Lab. Clin. Med.* **65**:179, 1965.
13. Heinemann HO, Fishman AP: Non-respiratory functions of mammalian lung. *Physiol. Reviews* **49**:1, 1969.
14. Hill JD, Osborn JJ, Swank RL, et al: Experience using a new Dacron wool filter during extracorporeal circulation. *Arch. Surg.* **101**:649, 1970.
15. Hirsch H, Swank RL, Breuer M, et al: Screen filtration pressure of homologous and heterologous blood and electroencephalogram. *Amer. J. Physiol.* **206**:811, 1964.
16. Hissen W, Swank RL: Screen filtration pressure and pulmonary hypertension. *Amer. J. Physiol.* **209**:715, 1965.
17. Jenevein Jr. EP, Weiss DL: Platelet microemboli associated with massive blood transfusion. *Amer. J. Path.* **45**:313, 1964.
18. Kartashevsky NG, Rumyantsev VV: Microclots of stabilized blood. *Probl. Gematol. Pereliv. Krovi* **13**:6 (**No. 5**) 1968.
19. Kattlove HE, Alexander B: The effect of cold on platelets. I. Cold-induced platelet aggregation. *Blood* **38**:39, 1971.
20. Kilduffe RA, DeBakey M: Methods and technique of transfusions. *In The Blood Bank and the Technique and Therapeutics of Transfusions.* St. Louis, Mo.: The C. V. Mosby Co., 1942, 370 pp.
21. Kolmer JA: Studies on the preservation of human blood. *Amer. J. Med. Sci.* **200**:311, 1940.
22. Kopriva CJ, Tobey RE, Herman CM, et al: The effect of hemorrhagic shock and massive transfusion on arterial oxygenation. *Ann. of Surg.,* in press, 1974.
23. LeVeen HH, Schatman B, Falk G: Polyolefin plastics as blood filters. *Surgery* **49**:510, 1961.
24. Lycette RM, Danforth WF, Koppel JL, et al: A new method for determining the size distribution of platelet aggregates. *Amer. J. Clin. Path.* **51**:445, 1969.
25. Mattern CFT, Brackett FS, Olson BJ: Determination of number and size of particles by electrical gating: Blood cells. *J. App. Physiol.* **10**:56, 1957.
26. Maycock WD, Mollison PL: A note on testing filters in blood transfusion sets. *Vox Sang.* **5**:157, 1960.
27. McCullough J, Benson SJ, Yanis EJ, et al: Effect of blood-bank storage on leukocyte function. *Lancet* **II**., 1333, 1969.

28. McNamara JJ, Burran EL, Suehiro G: Effective filtration of banked blood. *Surgery* **71**:594, 1972.
29. McNamara JJ, Molot MD, Strempie JF: Screen filtration pressure in combat casualties. *Ann Surg.* **172**:334, 1970.
30. McNamara JJ, Burran EL, Laeson E: Effect of debris in stored blood on pulmonary microvasculative. *Ann. Thorac. Surg.* **14**:133, 1972.
31. Moseley RV, Doty DB: Changes in the filtration characteristics of stored blood. *Ann. Surg.* **171**:329, 1970.
32. Moseley RV, Doty DB: Death associated with multiple pulmonary emboli soon after battle injury. *Ann. Surg.* **171**:336, 1970.
33. O'Brien JR: Platelet aggregation. Part II. Some results from a new method of study. *J. Clin. Path.* **15**:452, 1962.
34. Osborn JJ, Swank RL, Hill JD, et al: Clinical use of a Dacron wool filter during perfusion for open-heart surgery. *J. Thorac. Cardivasc. Surg.* **60**:575, 1970.
35. Patterson Jr. RH, Twichell JB: Disposable filter for microemboli. Use in cardiopulmonary bypass and massive transfusion. *J.A.M.A.* **215**:76, 1971.
36. Ruel, Jr. GJ, Greenburg SD, Lefrak EA, et al: Prevention of post-traumatic pulmonary insufficiency. Fine screen filtration of blood. *Arch. Surg.* **106**:386, 1973.
37. Shields CE: Evaluation of undefined material present in stored blood infusion. *Milit. Med.* **136**:351, 1971.
38. Shio H, Ramwell PW: Prostaglandin E_1 in platelet harvesting: An *in vitro* study. *Science* **175**:536, 1972.
39. Silver MJ: Platelet aggregation and plug formation: A model test system. *Amer. J. Physiol.* **218**:384, 1970.
40. Simmons RL, Heisterkamp III CA, Collins JA, et al: Respiratory insufficiency in combat casualties: IV. Hypoxemia during convalescence. *Ann. Surg.* **170**:53, 1969.
41. Solis RT, Gibbs MB: Filtration of the microaggregates in stored blood. *Transfusion* **12**:245, 1972.
42. Solis RT, Noon GP, DeBakey ME: Filtration characteristics of microemboli in stored and in autotransfused blood. *Trans. Amer. Soc. of Artif. Internal Organs,* in press, 1974.
43. Solis RT, Noon GP, Beall AC, et al: Particulate microembolization during cardiac operations. *Ann. Thorac. Surg.* **17**:332, 1974.
44. Solis RT, Goldfinger D, Gibbs MB, et al: Physical characteristics of microaggregates in stored blood. *Transfusion,* in press, 1974.

45. Swank RL: Alteration of blood on storage: Measurement of adhesiveness of "aging" platelets and leukocytes and their removal by filtration. *New Eng. J. Med.* **265**:723, 1961.
46. Swank RL: Platelet aggregation: Its role and cause in surgical shock. *J. Trauma* **8**:872, 1968.
47. Swank RL, Edwards MJ: Microvascular occlusion by platelet emboli after transfusion and shock. *Microvasc. Res.* **1**:15, 1968.
48. Swank RL, Porter GA: Disappearance of micro-emboli transfused into patients during cardiopulmonary bypass. *Transfusion* **3**:192, 1963.
49. Swank RL, Roth JG, Jansen J: Screen filtration pressure method and adhesiveness and aggregation of blood cells. *J. Appl. Physiol.* **19**:340, 1964.
50. Tullis L: Preservation of leukocytes. *Blood* **8**:563, 1953.
51. Walter CW, Bellamy Jr D, Murphy Jr WP: The mechanical factors responsible for rapid infusion of blood. *Surg. Gynecol. Obstet.* **101**:115, 1955
52. Walter CW, Button LN: Safe transfusion apparatus. *Anesthesiology* **27**:439, 1966.
53. Zeller JA, Gerard G, Gibbs MB, et al: An Electron Microscopic Study of Microaggregates in ACD Stored Blood. III Congress on Thrombosis and Haemostasis, Washington, D.C., p. 264, 1972.

THE EMILY COOLEY LECTURE
TRANSFUSION IN HISTORICAL PERSPECTIVE

Paul J. Schmidt

There is nothing new in the world except the history you do not know.

—TRUMAN

WE ARE doomed to repeat ourselves if we do not learn from history; in fact, if we do not learn from the preceding generation. In science, the generation span is short. For a young specialty like blood transfusion, the generation span is 15 years or less. Fifteen years is about the length of time that it takes for our new generation to do everything all over again: to rediscover old truths; to cloak old things in new language; and then to trumpet forth the good tidings with all the excitement due new findings.

In our science, the new worker's review of knowledge of the past is too often restricted to a skim of the index of the newest standard textbook. Any important work that is not cited in the standard text is presumed to not exist. The most recent current standard text in blood transfusion, dated 1972, contains slightly over 3,000 references.[14] One could expect, therefore, that it should contain the sum total of what is currently worth knowing. However, that 1972 textbook does not even refer to the Kilduffe and DeBakey book, the standard 1942 text which also contained 3,000 references, a summary of pre-World War II knowledge.[13] It can be argued that most of what we know about modern transfusion was learned after World War II. I agree, although with some reservations; but the 1972 text also does not refer to the 1949 book by Strumia and McGraw which showed the application of World War II knowledge to hospital practice.[19] In fact, the 1972 book does not reference the encyclopedic history by Kendrick of the World War II and Korean War experience which was published in 1964.[11] That history has another thousand references, almost all of them to unpublished materials in the National Research Council and the military files. You can say that was all 25 years ago. It was, but with the exception of blood component technology and hepatitis testing, there is little that most of us do that is different from what was done 25 years ago. The Kendrick volume makes my point most painfully. It decries over and over again how the military was slow to grasp the implications of transfusion in World War I, did not take advantage of the successful blood program of the Spanish Civil War, and ignored the

British experience of early World War II. Then, after we had finally evolved a blood program by 1945, the military junked that experience, and had to recreate everything anew for the Korean War.

So much for the textbook loss. We have another loser with us now, the computer search. Soon the uncritical searcher will accept the delusion that if some information is not in the computer printout, it does not exist. When that happens often enough, the 15-year generation span will be reduced. Poor programming, search loss, and file revision will all reduce memory to ten years, and then to five. You will soon find your neighbor repeating something you already did and published—soon you will be repeating yourselves.

It is to our own, as well as to the patient's and to the donor's advantage, that we learn from the past. All of us know of the apochryphal story of Pope Innocent VIII. He is supposed to have tried to regain his youth by taking the blood of young men. We are told that the young men died. In 1935, Bogdanof, Chief of the Moscow Transfusion Service, had a severe reaction after receiving 100 ml of blood from a young student. Both were of Group O, but evidently Bogdanof had been hyperimmunized. He had been the frequent recipient of such transfusions from young men. Put differently, he is said to have been "addicted" to transfusion. In this case, the old man died.[21]

I wish to point out some things we have learned, and can still learn, from achieving an historical perspective on transfusion. These things are mostly lessons from which someone in the past learned something —but from which there is much more to be gleaned. One has only to compare the 1652 method of Francis Potter (Fig. 1A)[22] with the 1919 apparatus of Brenizer (Fig. 1B[13]) to anticipate the 1953 plastic bag (Fig. 1C) as inevitable. We can only wonder why it took 300 years.

On Priority

The last 50 years of the 17th Century were the years of introduction of intravenous injections. From several places in Europe there were reports of the injection into the circulation of various solutions, including milk and wine and then blood. All of the interest was a natural outgrowth of the report of the discovery of the circulation by Harvey in 1628. It is always so; when the stage is set for logical exploitation of existing facts, new things will be done which are really applications of old knowledge with a new twist. The new things will probably be done in several places independently, wherever there are thinking men. All

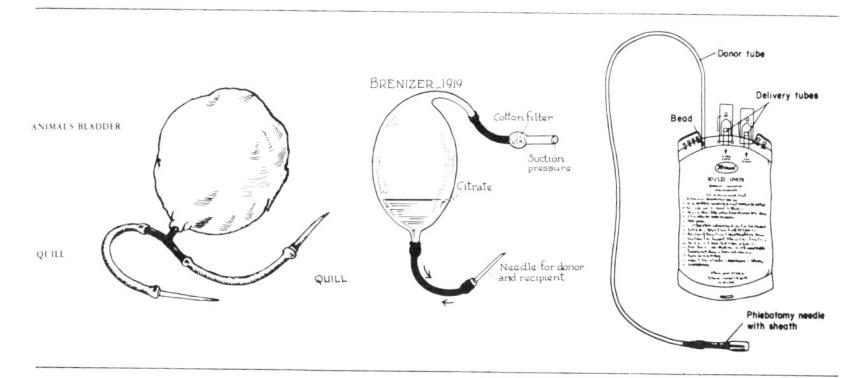

FIGURE 1A: Transfusion apparatus tried by Francis Potter in chickens, 1652.
FIGURE 1B: Citrated blood collection, 1919.
FIGURE 1C: Blood bag in original Fenwal® literature, July 1953.

of the interested parties have an exposure to the increased level of background knowledge, and all have been primed by the same circumstances to make the next logical step. In that way the first blood transfusions were described almost simultaneously by Denis in France and Lower in England, with a few other contestants in other parts of Europe. Here then, with the first stories of transfusion, we also find the first arguments about priority. The argument revolves, like so many of the priority problems today, on delays in publication. There are only two copies of the transfusion journal of that day, *The Philosophical Transactions of the Royal Society of London,* which are dated *July* 1667 and contain Denis' letter on the first transfusion of man with animal blood. That issue of the journal was promptly suppressed and later was reissued with a date of *September* 1667. The reason given by the editor, Henry Oldenburg, was that he was required to desist from publication in July because of an "extraordinary accident." The excuse was a good one because the "extraordinary accident" actually consisted of his incarceration in the Tower of London on charges of high treason.[12] When Oldenburg was found innocent, he returned to the wars of debate on who was first, Denis or Lower. Despite many nasty comments of the day on who did what first, it is accepted today that Denis does have the priority for the first human transfusions.

I am sure that most of the scientists, and all of the editors here, have had a similar event happen to them. It isn't that anybody has stolen our ideas, it is just that the world was ready for that piece of information to be found and reported, and somebody else got it into print first. An illustration of the compounding of the priority battles is the statement in the foreword to *Advances in Blood Grouping,* Vol. III, by Wiener. He tells us that his book entitled *Blood Groups and Transfusion,* appeared in 1932, before the classic books of Schiff and Steffan, and before the English translation of Lattes. However, although Wiener's book is really the first modern book on the subject, when I checked the actual publication date it was not 1932, but only after those others, i.e. in 1935. What is the answer? The material was ready for publication in 1932 but was delayed for three years by the publisher.[23] Under those circumstances, many people wish that they too could consign some editors to the Tower of London.

When the transfusion story cropped up again in the literature 150 years later, the priority battles were reentered. This time it was not France vs. England, but with the new spirit of independence, it was America First! There is a footnote in a Philadelphia journal issued in 1825 which reports on Blundell's work but says, "Thirty years ago, the experiment of transfusion of blood under precisely the same circumstances as above, was performed by Dr. Physick."[7] The details of Philip Syng Physick's transfusion experience have eluded confirmation. Is it true? Was the first human to human blood transfusion given in America? Or, was the report just American chauvinism? Of course the issue is not important in human history. There is no doubt that Blundell, the Englishman, really did the first scientific and physiological studies of human transfusion. Nevertheless, patents have been issued and fortunes have been made on less evidence than what was contained in that footnote about Physick.

Hopefully, these historical vignettes on priority will provide some solace for those who will be "scooped" tomorrow on work that they did yesterday.

On Regulation

There is yet more to be learned from Denis' first experience with transfusion. It has to do with governmental rule and regulation. The usual story that we hear is that after the first malpractice suit for transfusion, Denis was enjoined in 1667 from ever transfusing again, and transfusion was banned by a Church and State edict. Not so! Denis took pains to point out in 1668 that he had been found not guilty of malpractice, and that transfusion was not actually prohibited. The only verdict was that future transfusions should be performed under the authority of the proper regulatory body, in his case the

Medical Faculty of Paris.[9] In practice it must be admitted that the end result was the same. At the same time that we had the first human transfusion, we had the first biologics control, the first regulatory body, the first minimum requirements. The fact that the French regulatory agency proceeded to deliberate transfusion for so long that it was not used for 150 years was an incidental, although ominous, portent of things to come.

Another interesting story has now surfaced with the publication of a new history of the U. S. Public Health Service by Furman, who worked from unpublished documents in the National Library of Medicine.[8] She tells why the Biologics Control Act of 1902 was a complete surprise to the regulators, although later on they took full credit for it. The law, as many of you know, began as a local bill for the District of Columbia in a reaction to a tetanus scare in the production of smallpox vaccine in horses. Furman tells us that when the bill was about to fail for lack of interest, a physician in the District took advantage of his strategic professional position on the last day of that session. He had, as his personal patients, the four men needed to get the bill passed: The Vice President, the Speaker of the House, and the chairmen of both the Senate and the House committees on legislation for the District of Columbia. He telephoned them all. He asked each presiding officer to recognize the chairman of his District of Columbia committee when he would stand up. Then he asked each chairman to ask for recognition from the floor. It was so done, and by that skillful maneuver in medical politics, the bill was sent on to Teddy Roosevelt by acclamation from both Houses of Congress; and we had federal biologics control.

Most of you know some of the later history of that law. You have been told that the federal government logically accepted blood products for licensing under the 1902 Act. That interpretation was challenged in the courts in 1962 and the government finally won the case on grounds that human plasma was always included in the "plain meaning" of the law, as supported by "purpose, administrative construction, and legislative history."[20] What was the real story?

Plasma was first taken out of the hospital laboratory for large scale pooling and processing in the "Plasma for Britain" program of the Blood Transfusion Betterment Association in New York City, the lineal ancestor of the New York Blood Center. In his final report, Dr. Charles R. Drew, the Medical Director of that program, describes a meeting on September 25, 1940 among their legal counsel and the

Federal, State, and City authorities. There they received the ruling by the National Institute of Health that the plasma program was not subject to the federal laws regulating biologic products.[2]

Later in that same year, Dr. Edwin Cohn began his first labors to produce a beef albumin for injection into humans. It is not generally appreciated that the Cohn fractionation methods, still the standard process for blood fractionation today, had their beginnings in an attempt to make a despeciated crystaline beef albumin suitable for use in humans. Almost invariably every one will remember the age-old goal: use of animal blood in humans. They are surprised that it was Cohn's major scientific endeavor up until 1942—it is of course still being pursued for the preparation of animal Factor VIII. Let me remind you of the recent use of bovine red cells in the famous paper on the discovery of blood group I by Wiener in 1956. That title tells the story, **"Type Specific Cold Auto-Antibodies as a Cause of Acquired Hemolytic Anemia and Hemolytic Reactions: Biologic Test with Bovine Red Cells."** Cohn spent two years without achieving his goal. Perhaps they were not lost years. They did lay the groundwork for human

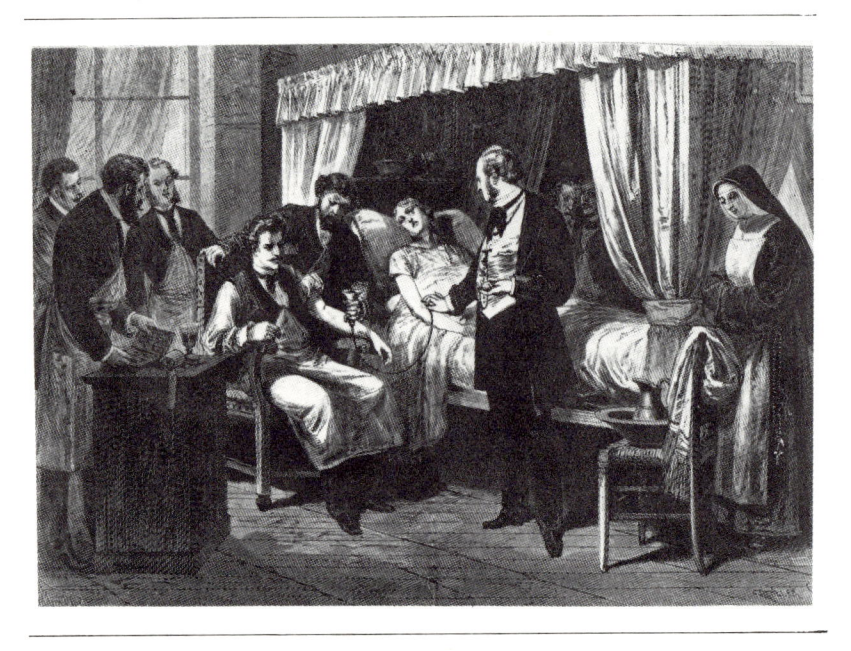

FIGURE 2: Paris transfusion, Harper's Weekly, July 1874. (Courtesy of National Library of Medicine)

plasma fractionation and they did result in the National Institute of Health going into the human blood and plasma business. Despite its September, 1940 disclaimer of jurisdiction over plasma, the government published its first blood rules, the Minimum Requirements for Unfiltered Normal Human Plasma, on 20 February 1941. It had reversed itself in five months, with a speed probably unmatched since then. Perhaps there are parallels among the tetanus-in-horses scare, the pressure on the National Institute of Health to enter into the field of biologics control, and now the National Blood Policy built on the hepatitis scare. Perhaps some time in the future it can be determined whether such regulations, established under scare pressure, are always beneficial.

On Technique

Before 1900, transfusion was done so infrequently that no expertise in technique was available. The procedure was a medical curiosity as pictured in Harper's Weekly (Fig. 2), and photographed at Bellevue

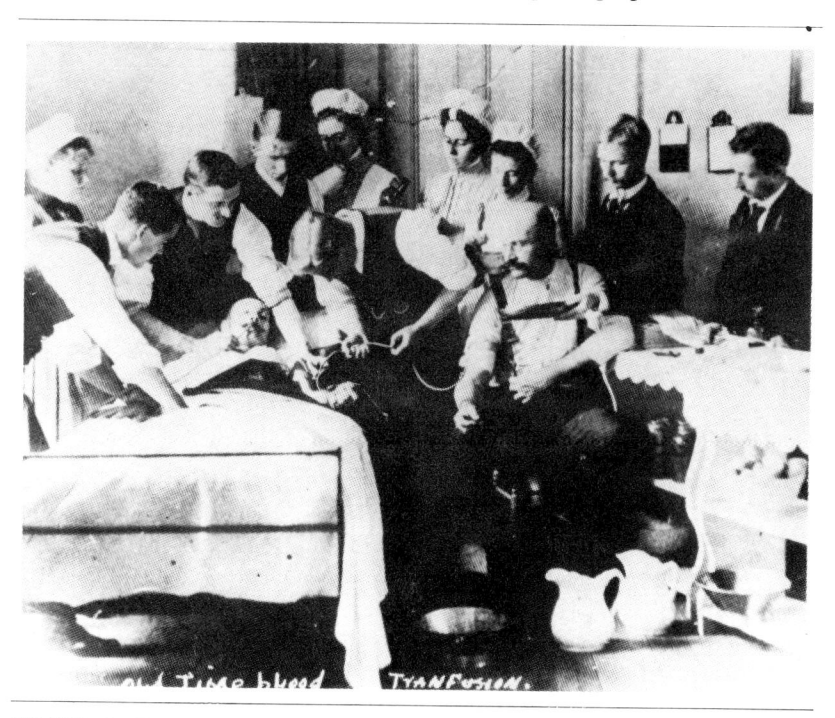

FIGURE 3: Direct transfusion at Bellevue Hospital around 1880. (Courtesy of Dr. William J. Kuhns)

(Fig. 3). Then, in the first 15 years of this century, just as in the last 50 years of the 17th Century, everything happened at once. Because Landsteiner discovered the ABO blood groups in 1900, and Crile published his cannula method for direct transfusion in 1907, and Ottenberg popularized crossmatching beginning in 1908, one tends to assume that the events occurred in a logical sequence, one based upon the other. Not so! Crile rejected Landsteiner's ideas on hemagglutination and immunity, and Ottenberg's first transfusion was performed with no blood grouping or compatibility testing. The total disregard of the practitioner for Landsteiner's findings is well described by Bernheim, one of the early surgical transfusionists.[1] A reading of his report of the controversy over the importance of the ABO groups as related to red cell transfusion is a remarkable parallel to the controversy about HL-A groups and platelet transfusion today: Are the groups important? What is the best test? Why are there failures despite test predictions? What is a crossmatch? Are we really drawing scientific conclusions, or are they prejudiced impressions?

Crile of Cleveland published his epic book, the first American monograph on transfusion, two years after his cannula paper, that is, in 1909.[4] He was still ignoring Landsteiner, although he had a respect for a hemolysin test that took two days to perform. If the donor's serum hemolyzed the recipient's cells, he thought that there was reason to proceed carefully. The constituents of his test, donor's serum and patient's cells, were what we would call the *minor* crossmatch, but even then Crile did not accept that hemolysis was due to genetic differences. Like some researchers of today, Crile attempted to make a test for cancer out of his observations. He concluded that the red cells were destroyed by some toxic process inherent in the recipient and activated by the influx of donor serum. On the other hand, if the recipient's serum hemolyzed the donor's red cells in his test, in a manner similar to today's major crossmatch, that was *not* a contraindication to transfusion. Furthermore, he says, "Agglutination of the red corpuscles and precipitation may also occur, but, from a patient standpoint at least, the author has had no reason to believe that these two last changes may be regarded as probable sources of danger." Small wonder that with his approach, plus the manipulation of the blood vessels in a field of questionable sterility, and doused in mineral oil and pyrogenic saline, and despite the liberal use of morphine, Crile found that the febrile reaction was "expected and usually occurs."

Early in this century, blood transfusion developed as a recognized surgical specialty. The 1928 book editor of the *American Journal of*

Surgery wrote: "One may almost assert that a homo medico cannot aspire to immortality in the surgical realm unless he has devised and has called after his name a blood-transfusion apparatus."[3] Perhaps some of the enmity between blood bankers and surgeons is because we have invaded their domain. Perhaps we should say rather that we have accepted their leftovers. Please remember that the "wal" in Fenwal derives from the name of Carl Walter, a surgeon, and that Richard Lewisohn, whose citrate method freed us evenually from the "direct" transfusion, was also a surgeon. Nevertheless, for the first 40 years of this century, the regular use of preserved, liquid blood was still in the future, and there was no "blood banking" as we know it today. "Direct" transfusion required placing the donor and the patient in juxtaposition and providing some means of propelling the blood in the right direction, i.e. from donor to recipient, and hopefully not the reverse. Of course the whole procedure could be upsetting to both donor and recipient. The biographer of Joseph Goldberger tells of the direct transfusions given in 1928 to that eminent physician, "He didn't want to know whose blood he was taking—until afterward; he kept a towel over his face during the transfusions; it stirred him too much to think that this pal or that son was giving his blood to him."[15]

Between 1915 and 1940, a large number of direct transfusion instruments were made and sold. In the words of Scannell, one of the most famous New York transfusionists, "Any one who expects to do blood transfusion should not only own, but also take personal care of his apparatus."[18] Crile had put it another way in 1909, "transfusion is a problem in mechanics as well as therapeutics." Some of the pieces of apparatus, like that of Kiernan (Fig. 4), were themselves complex mechanical marvels; others, like that of Aveling, were extremely simple (Fig. 5). There were those that proved to have lasting scientific and practical value.

Equipment

1. *Direct Artery to Vein Connections.*

In 1907, Crile invented tiny cannulas which were used to connect donor and patient (Fig. 6). The method entailed the actual joining of an artery of the donor to a vein of the recipient. That highly skilled performance required the most precise approximation of the blood vessels to permit flow, and to prevent clotting. It also required a permanent sacrifice of the artery of the donor. If the operation was successful, the donor's blood, under its higher arterial pressure, would be

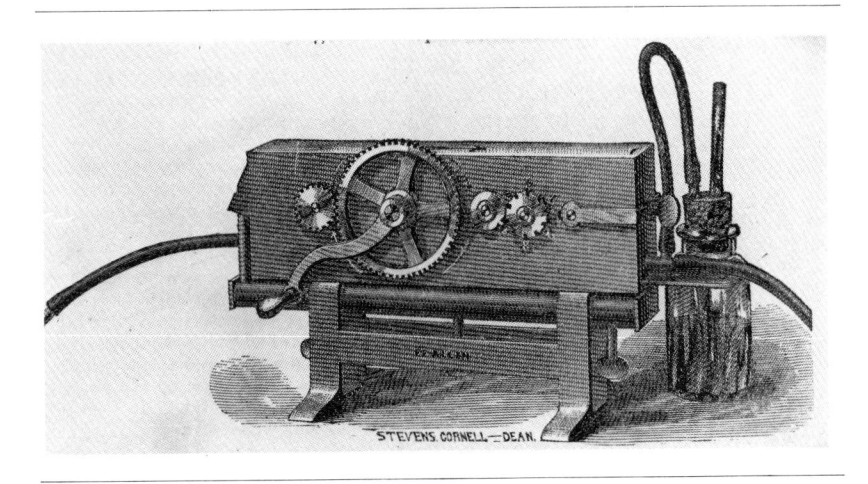

FIGURE 4: Kiernan-Allen roller pump. (From Kiernan: Chicago Medical Review, 1882)

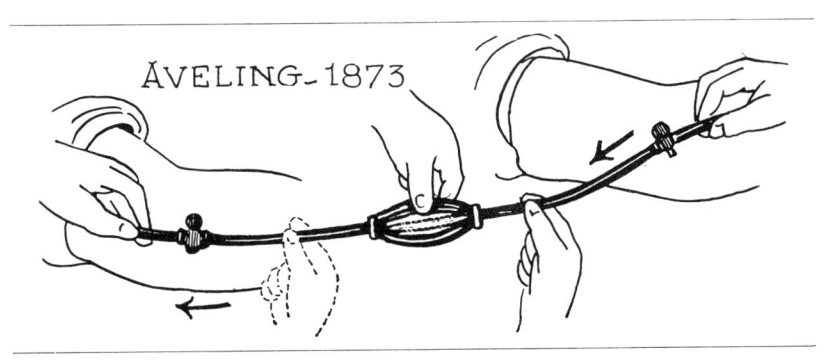

FIGURE 5: Aveling squeeze bulb apparatus. (From Kilduffe and DeBakey: The Blood Bank and the Technique and Therapeutics of Transfusions. St. Louis, 1942, C. V. Mosby Co.)

forced into the recipient's vein. The transfusion was continued until the donor fainted or the patient seemed to be improved. Since there was no way to measure the actual flow (and there might be none going on if a clot had formed), the rules were arbitrary. Crile's rule was that "enough blood must be transfused to accomplish as much good as possible, and yet too much must not be given." In his book he reports on anastomoses which were continued for between 8 and 80 minutes, but the majority were for about 30 minutes. One of his greatest problems was circulatory overload in the patient, and another was collapse

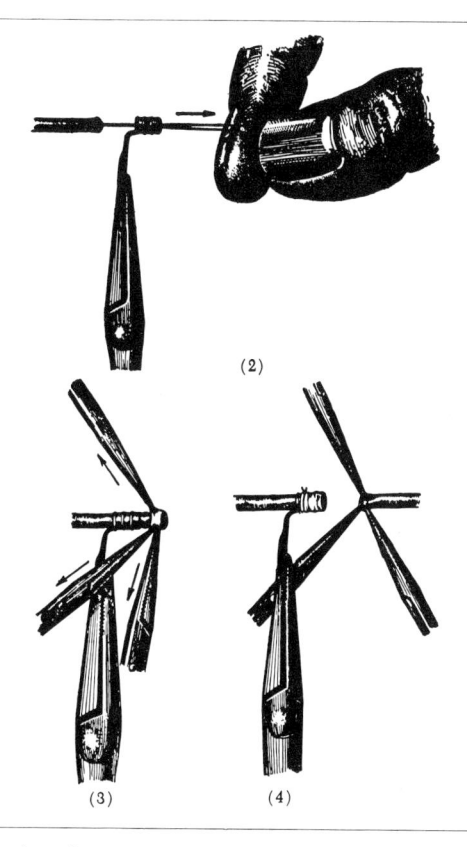

FIGURE 6: Artery to vein anastomosis with Crile cannula, 1907.

of the donor, so we can assume that those were large, as well as rapid, transfusions.

Crile states that in his large series, he used paid donors only twice. He did have a problem with some potential voluntary donors whom he describes as having "a certain amount of distrust of both surgeons and hospitals." One of his donors was hooked up to a patient for 56 minutes and was about to faint, but was revived by pouring cold water on his abdomen. After an hour's rest, he walked upstairs to be weighed and there he collapsed, nauseated, faint and perspiring. He was revived again, this time with extremity bandages and strychnine. The donor had lost four pounds, which might have consisted of the blood, sweat, and tears from that episode. Since it was mostly blood, that would be the equivalent of a four unit bleeding by today's standards.

Crile also did exchange transfusions and used the inflatable pneumatic suits rediscovered lately and now called a spin-off of today's space technology. He describes one case as follows: "Before the transfusion was begun, the patient's lower extremities were placed in a rubber pneumatic suit. He was then gradually bled of 1,400 ml. As this was done, the suit was slowly inflated, and he was lowered more and more into the head-down position to prevent cerebral and cardiac anemia during the bleeding." In another case he tells us of the whole problem of his method. He first bled one of his intended recipients of 1600 ml and tells us that the patient had "marked depression, wrinkling of the face, pallor, free perspiration, running pulse, restlessness and air-hunger." After all of that, the anastomosis could not be made because the donor was then found to have an aberrant double radial artery. All in all, the anastomosis system was impractical, transfusions were used only in extremis, and the donor not only lost an artery, but also might end up sewn to a patient who had died during the process.

2. *Syringe Transfer Using Special Needles*

In 1892, von Ziemssen had tried a "bucket brigade" process in which large needles were placed into the veins (or sometimes arteries) of the donor and the recipient. One surgeon would draw a small amount of blood into a syringe through a special needle fixed in the donor, disconnect the syringe, and then pass it quickly to a second operator who would inject the needle fixed in the recipient. Each syringe of blood was followed by an injection of saline into the patient to prevent clotting in that needle. Meanwhile, the first surgeon was drawing another syringe from the donor and an assistant was washing out each syringe in turn with water, and passing more syringes to the first operator. The method was made popular by Lindeman who began his transfusion career as a Bellevue intern in 1913 (Fig. 7). The procedure required a highly practiced team to repeat the process over and over again as rapidly as possible. Many such transfers were needed to give one pint of blood. The donor lost a lot more, since his tourniquet was left on between syringe changes, and, inevitably, blood covered the floor and all of the participants. Attempts were made to keep the blood from clotting in the syringes and needles by coating them internally with mineral oil and paraffin.

3. *Syringe and Stopcock*

A combination of methods one and two was introduced in 1911 by Curtis and David of Chicago.[5] They described an elongated Crile can-

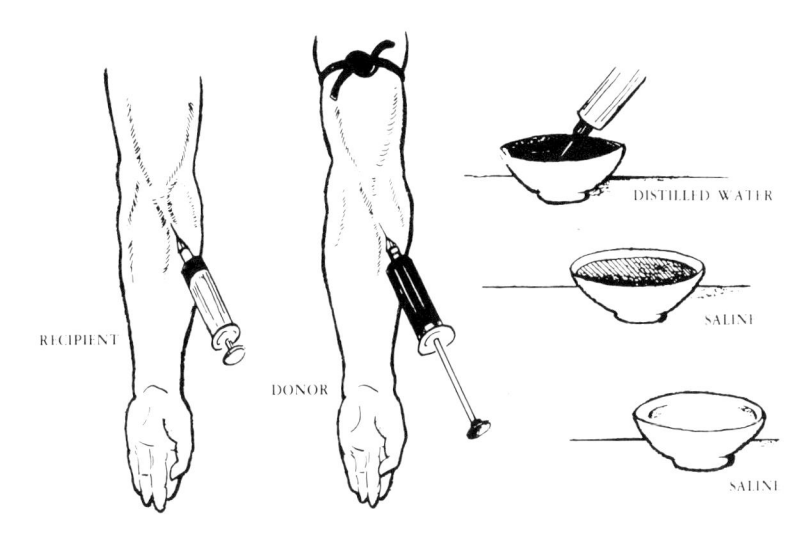

LINDEMANN - MULTIPLE SYRINGE METHOD - 1913

FIGURE 7: Multiple syringe method.

nula (Fig. 8) which had a joint in it where a syringe was attached. Their clear purpose was both to propel the blood and to measure the volume transfused. With their system, it was no longer necessary to sacrifice a donor artery with each transfusion, and vein to vein transfusion became the method of choice. However, their inflexible apparatus was soon improved; the cannulae became needles and tubing, and the popular Unger appartus was introduced in 1915 (Fig. 9). The needles were again placed in donor and in recipient, but were now connected to each other through a valve and double syringe arrangement. Blood was drawn from the donor and into one syringe through the valve, while saline was being injected into the recipient from the other syringe. The valve was then turned so that when the blood syringe was emptied into the recipient, saline was flushing the donor path.

The process was repeated as often as was necessary to transfer the desired amount, or until either the donor or the patient had an adverse reaction. The tubing, valves and syringe had to be kept small to reduce the danger of clotting in the system. Sometimes a clot would freeze the system and blood would spurt all over the room. Unger's stopcock

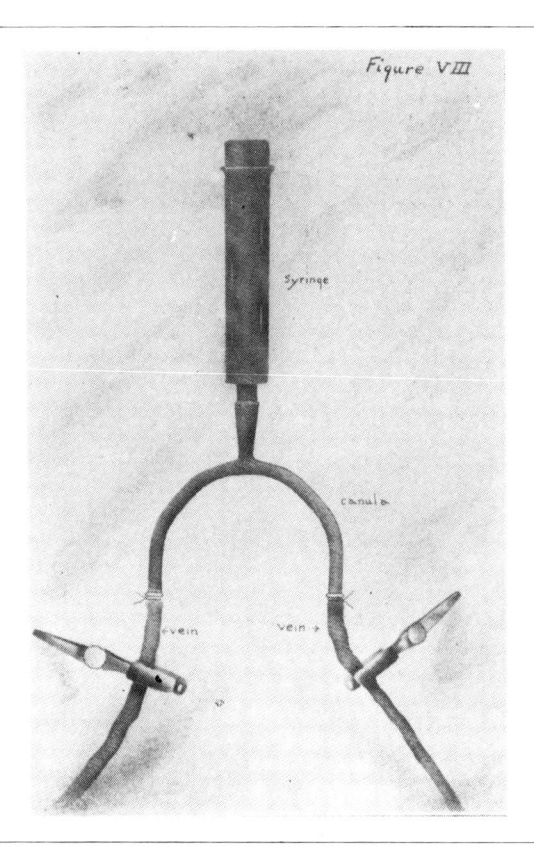

FIGURE 8: Curtis-David cannula with syringe attached for vein to vein transfusion, 1911. (From Winthrop: South. Med. J. 1911)

had dead space which could pass some of the recipient's blood to the donor and, like all of the other systems before it, required at least two highly skilled operators. The dead space in Unger's instrument was eliminated by Tzanck in 1926 with a syringe which moved as the valve, eliminating valve space (Fig. 10). The popular Scannell apparatus permitted the syringe to be held, and the stopcock to be turned, all with the same hand (Fig. 11). An automatic ball-valve system which would shunt the flow was developed by Soresi in 1925 on the principle of the old Potain syringe (Fig. 12). However, the automatic reversal apparatuses had faults: clotting in the shunt system, or recipient hypertension, could reverse the entire flow. When that happened, the operator would begin to transfuse from patient to donor, with no warning. Finally, the simple DeBakey-Gillentine sleeve valve was developed in

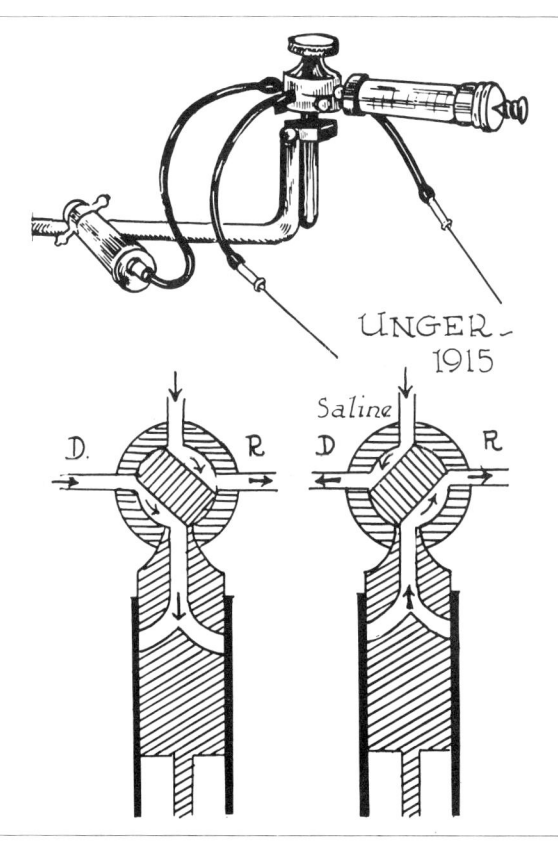

FIGURE 9: Unger four-way stopcock. (From Kilduffe and DeBakey; C. V. Mosby Co.)

New Orleans in 1932, and the simplest became the best (Fig. 13).

4. *Roller Pump*

It was hoped that there would be less trauma to the blood, and less clotting, if the flow path was as regular as possible. Attempts to milk the transfusion tubing, instead of relying on the pumping action of the donor's heart, or on syringes, had been suggested as early as 1876. The DeBakey roller pump (1934) was the epitome of the method (Fig. 14). A rubber tube which went from donor needle to recipient needle was "milked" by a rotating roller, turned by hand. The tubing could be kept small and lined with mineral oil to retard clotting. The apparatus solved the problem of the "creeping" of the tubing through the rollers, and it had an automatic counter which showed the number

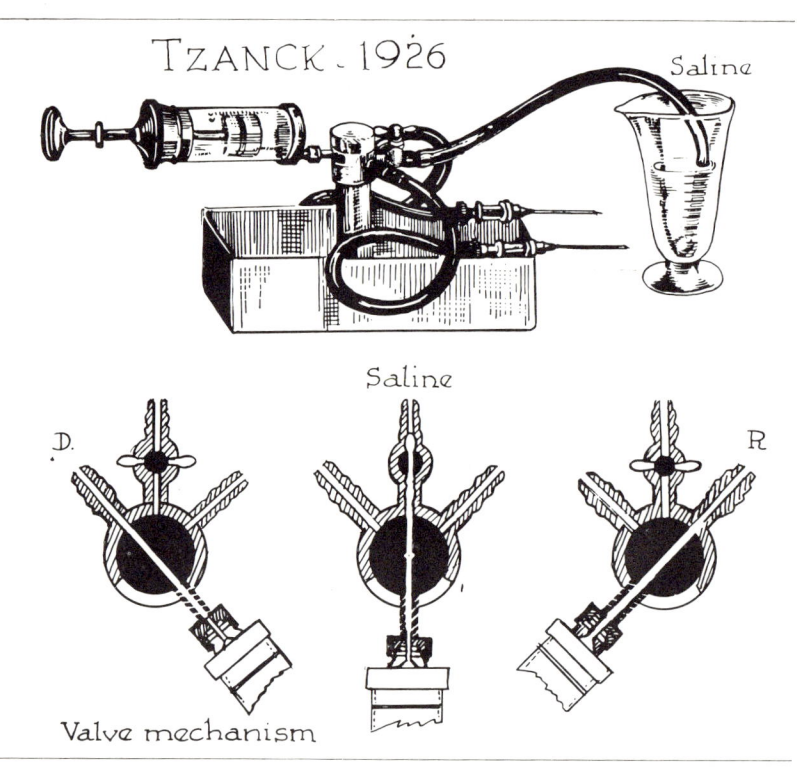

FIGURE 10: Three-way stopcock method (From Kilduffe and DeBakey; C. V. Mosby Co.)

of roller revolutions. Each revolution of a roller meant one milliliter transfused. There was an automatic lock to prevent turning the rollers the wrong way.

The genius of DeBakey, who began his surgical career as a transfusionist, was that he perfected the best system in 1932, the sleeve valve, and then that he was able to discard it in 1934 for something better, the roller pump. However, with the advent of the post World War II blood bank as we know it today, the roller pump was never fully appreciated for transfusion. Then, in 1953, Gibbon performed the first successful surgery employing total cardiopulmonary bypass. He used DeBakey pumps in his oxygenator system, and, again in the hands of a surgeon, the transfusion pump achieved its greatest importance.[10]

5. *Citrate-Syringe Methods*

Sodium citrate anticoagulant had been used extensively since Lewi-

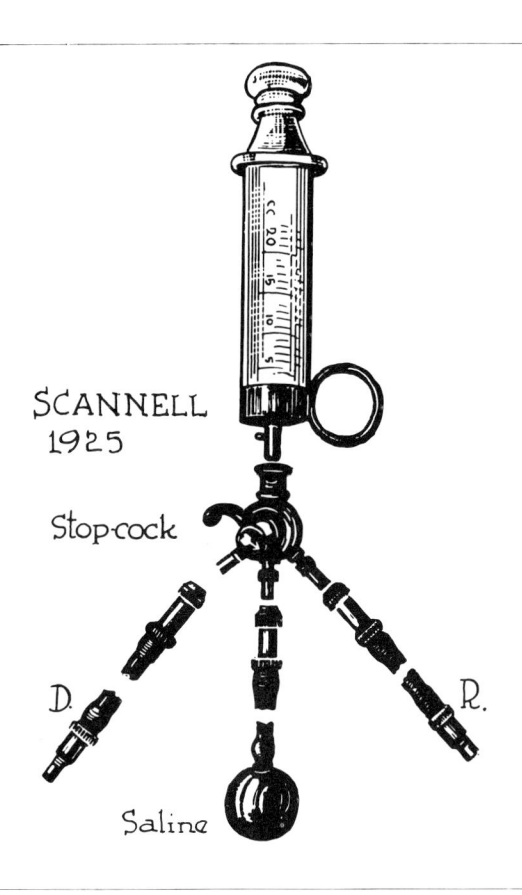

FIGURE 11: Compact three-way stopcock and syringe. (From Kilduffe and DeBakey; C. V. Mosby Co.)

sohn popularized it in 1915 (Fig. 15). However, early citrated blood transfusions caused fever and chills in half of the recipients. It was later proved, of course, that the ill effect was due not to the citrate itself, but was due to bacterial pyrogens in the water used to make the citrate solution. With that problem solved, "indirect" transfusion became the method of choice during the Spanish Civil War and World War II. In an interesting transitional system, the three-way stopcock method was combined with the citrate method. A syringe had been invented by Jube in 1924 which had a groove in the barrel (Fig. 16). When the barrel was turned from the port which led to the donor to the one which led to recipient, the groove acted as an internal stop-

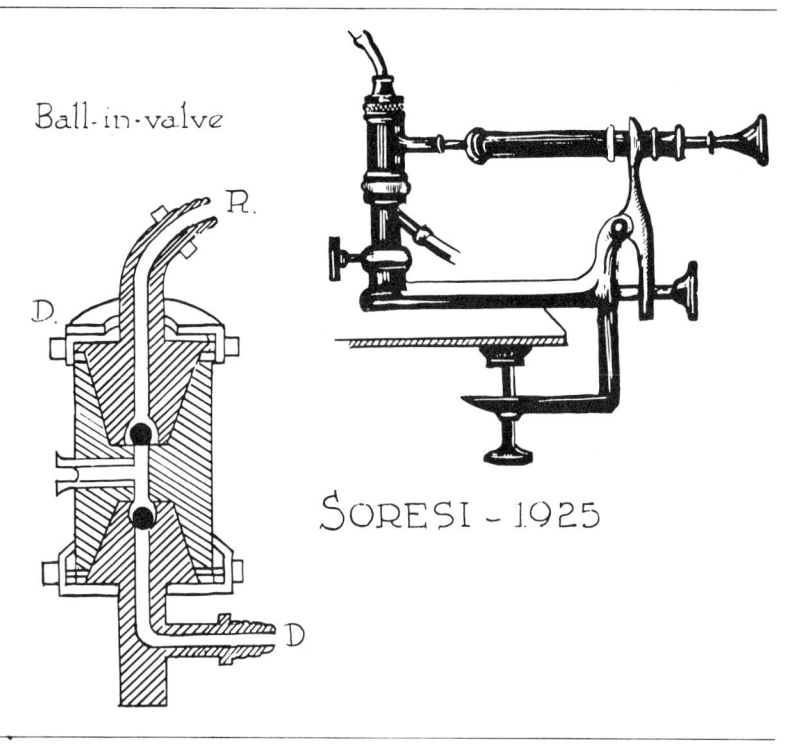

FIGURE 12: Automatic ball-valve stopcock and syringe. (From Kilduffe and DeBakey; C. V. Mosby Co.)

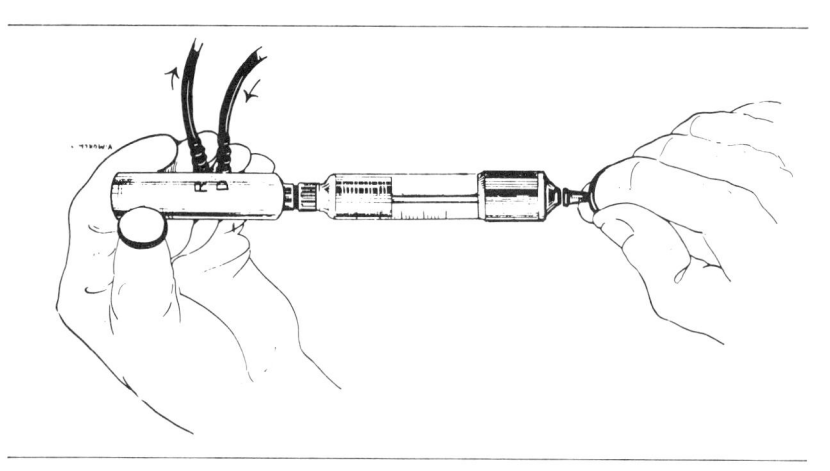

FIGURE 13: Sleeve-valve method of DeBakey and Gillentine. (From Kilduffe and DeBakey; C. V. Mosby Co.)

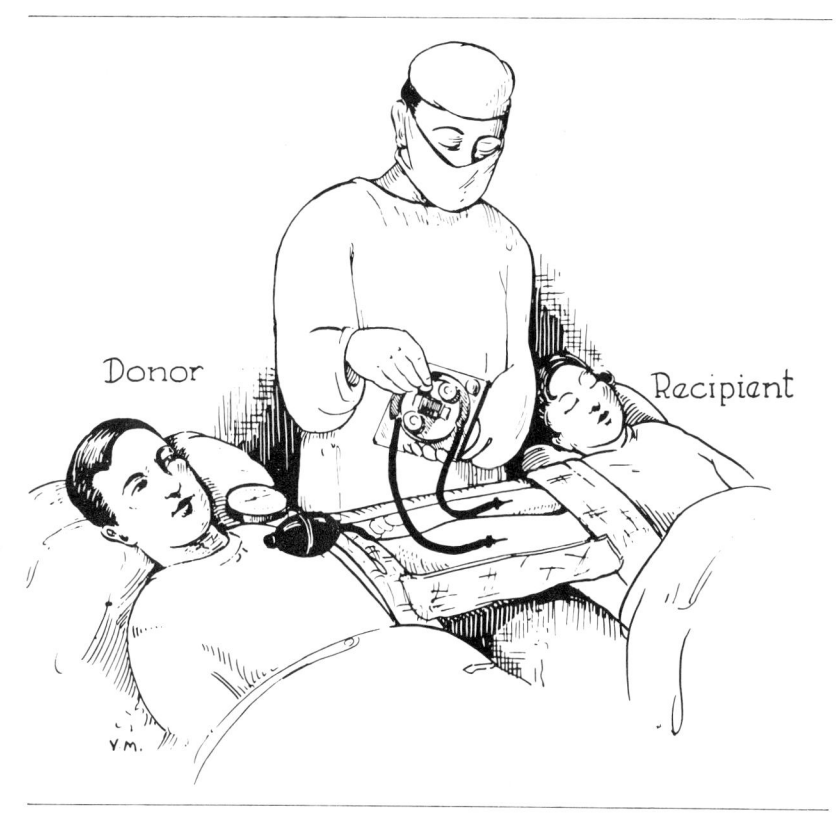

FIGURE 14: DeBakey rotary pump in use; note direction of donor needle. (From Kilduffe and DeBakey; C. V. Mosby Co.)

cock. The idea was improved by Goepel in 1932 to provide for a third port for saline (which was delivered from a sterile male urinal). In the elegant "Medical Center" set,[6] citrate solution was kept in the reservoir over the syringe. Each turn of the syringe barrel also permitted a few drops of anticoagulant to enter the sytem. The apparatus, fitted with counters and locks, was sold by Becton-Dickinson from 1933 to 1941. It was in use for ten years after that by those who had enough skill and enough practice to be able to manage the complex assembly and operation.

6. *Exchange Transfusion of the Newborn*

When Rh hemolytic disease of the newborn (erythroblatosis fetalis) was recognized in the 1940's, exchange transfusion soon proved to be lifesaving treatment. In order to remove and replace blood in those

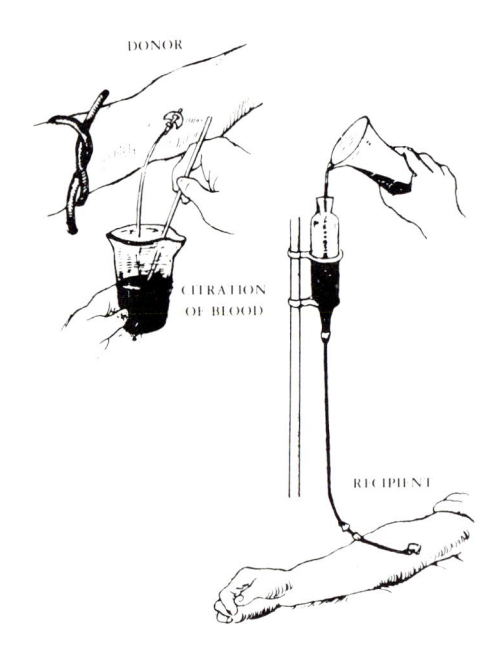

LEWISOHN - CITRATE TRANSFUSION
1915

FIGURE 15: The first practical citrate method: note direction of donor needle.

tiny recipients, pumping methods again became necessary. Rosenfield[17] has pointed out that the whole story of the evolution of transfusion technique was repeated again for this special purpose. The Tzanck modification of the Unger apparatus reappeared.[16] Lindeman-type needles were reintroduced. The optimum stopcock method of Allen and Diamond depended on the then new polyethylene tubing (Figs. 17, 18). The original equipment employed tandem three-way stopcocks and the Allen needle (a cannula fitted to plastic tubing).

On the Future

Crile tells us in italics in the last sentence in his book: "Judiciously employed, transfusion will surely prove a valuable, often life-saving, resource; injudiciously employed, it will surely become discredited."

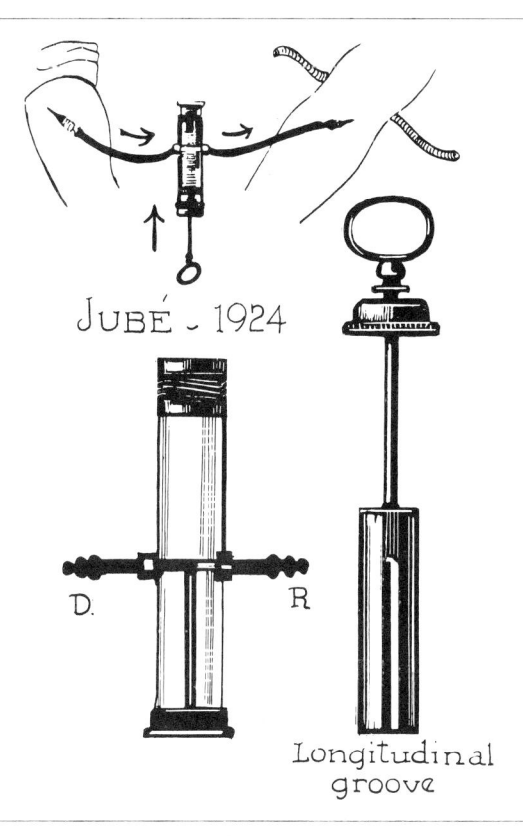

FIGURE 16: Syringe with groove barrel valve. (From Kilduffe and DeBakey; C. V. Mosby Co.)

Today, 65 years later, blood is considered valuable, and life-saving. It has even been declared by an ex-President to be a "national" resource. All of us can remember some injudicious uses of transfusion which have been discredited and which have almost discredited the whole field of endeavor. It is only with an appreciation of the ground that we have been over that we can approach the best path of the future.

What is the goal of the future? The goal of the future is to put ourselves out of business. Transfusion therapy is only substitution therapy. We are already returning to the management of acute blood loss without transfusion; isoimmunization due to pregnancy is being prevented; exchange transfusion of the newborn is becoming less frequent. In the laboratory, red cells can be coaxed to carry and release oxygen on demand, and the production of specific blood components may be pos-

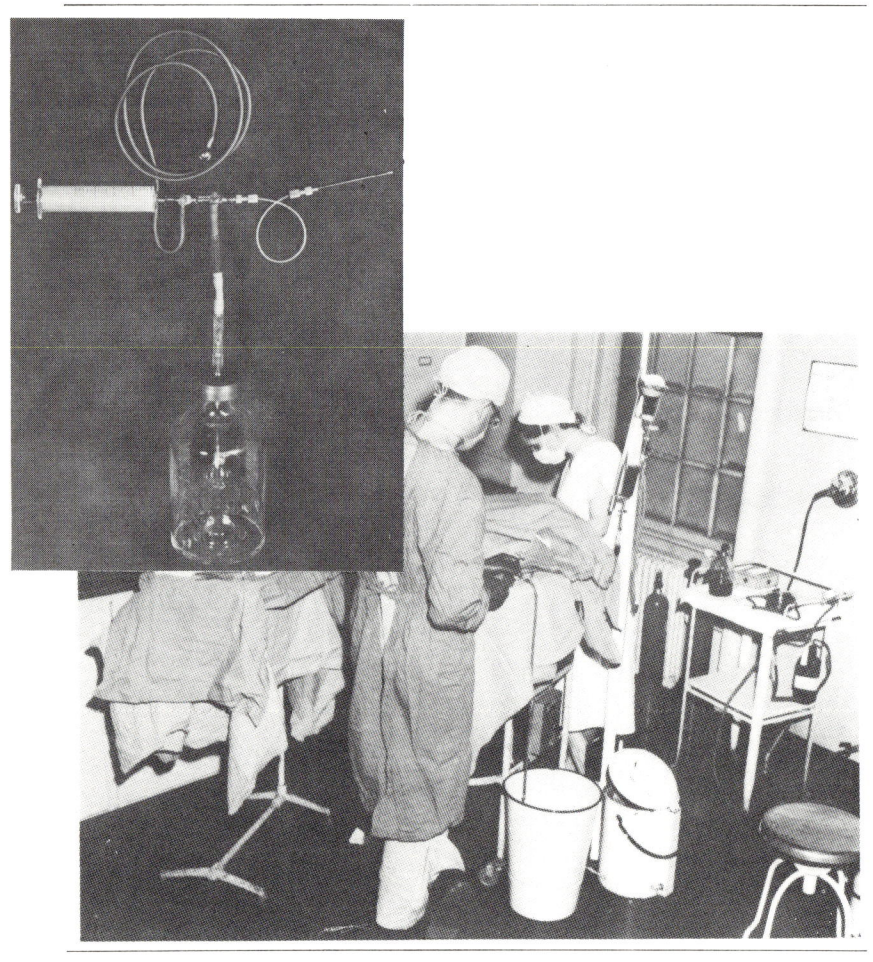

FIGURE 17: Allen and Diamond apparatus for exchange transfusion of the newborn. (Courtesy of Dr. Louis K. Diamond)

FIGURE 18: Exchange transfusion of the newborn, around 1947. (Courtesy of Dr. Louis K. Diamond)

sible in tissue culture. In the patient, we expect that the chronic deficiencies of blood components will be repaired by the transplantation of specific generative tissues. Each such step of tomorrow depends on what we are learning today, but depends also on what we have learned from yesterday. Study the past, or you will have to repeat it all again.

REFERENCES

1. Bernheim BM: *Adventure in Blood Transfusion.* New York: Smith & Durrell, 1942, 182 pp.
2. Blood Transfusion Association: *Narrative Account of Work and Medical Report.* New York: Blood Transfusion Association, 1941, 121 pp.
3. Book Review: *Am. J. Surg.* **IV**:243, 1928.
4. Crile GW: *Hemorrhage and Transfusion.* New York: D. Appleton, 1909, 560 pp.
5. Curtis AM, David VC: Transfusion of blood by a new method, allowing accurate measurement. *JAMA* **56**:35, 1911.
6. Dutton WF, Lake GB: *Parenteral Therapy.* Springfield: CC Thomas, 1936, 386 pp.
7. Transfusion of blood. *Phila. J. Med. Phys. Sci.* **9**:205, 1825.
8. Furman B: *A Profile of the United States Public Health Service, 1798-1948.* USDHEW Publication No. (NIH) 73-369, 1973, 487 pp.
9. Hall AR: English medicine in the Royal Society's correspondence: 1660-1677. *Med. Hist.* **XV**: 111, 1971.
10. Hewitt RL, Creech O, Jr: History of the pump oxygenator. *Arch. Surg.* **93**:680, 1966.
11. Kendrick DB: *Blood Program in World War II.* Washington: Office of the Surgeon General, Department of the Army, 1964, 922 pp.
12. Keynes G: Tercentenary of blood transfusion. *Br. Med. J.* **4**:410, 1967.
13. Kilduffe RA, DeBakey M: *The Blood Bank and the Technique and Therapeutics of Transfusions.* St. Louis: C. V. Mosby, 1942, 558 pp.
14. Mollison PL: *Blood Transfusion in Clinical Medicine.* Oxford: Blackwell, Ed. 5, 1972, 830 pp.
15. Parsons RP: *Trail to Light, A Biography of Joseph Goldberger.* Indianapolis: Bobbs-Merrill Co., 1943, 353 pp.
16. Pollak OJ: Personal communication.
17. Rosenfield RE: Early twentieth century origins of modern blood transfusion therapy. *Mt. Sinai J. Med.* **41**:625, 1974.
18. Scannell JM: Blood transfusion. *Am. J. Surg.* **36**:26, 1937.

19. Strumia MM, McGraw JJ: *Blood and Plasma Transfusions*. Philadelphia: F. A. Davis Company, 1949, 497 pp.
20. U. S. Court of Appeals, Second Circuit, Docket No. 28498, Brief for the United States of America.
21. Vlados C, Meerson J: Les reactions graves et les complications mortelles consecutives a la transfusion du sang. *Le Sang.* **9**:375, 1935.
22. Webster C: The origins of blood transfusion: A reassessment. *Med. Hist.* **XV**:387, 1971.
23. Wiener AS: Personal communication.

ACKNOWLEDGEMENT: I wish to thank Drs. Michael DeBakey, Louis Diamond, O. J. Pollak and Leon Sussman who contributed equipment and information; Dr. DeBakey for permission to use illustrations from his book, and Dr. Richard Rosenfield for a preprint of his current work.

DISEASES TRANSMITTED BY BLOOD TRANSFUSION
Harold A. Oberman

IN THE ensuing discussion we will concern ourselves with those conditions in which the donor blood contains organisms which do not necessarily result in an immediate adverse effect in the recipient, but later may produce manifestations of the corresponding disease. Although viral hepatitis continues to assume major importance in this respect, especially in the United States, the growth of world travel during the past decade has increased the need for awareness of other conditions which may be transmitted by this route.

It should be recognized that any pathogenic organism in the blood stream of the donor is capable of producing disease in the recipient. However, the fragility of the organism, especially on storage at 4 C in citrate, as well as the defense mechanisms of the recipient, may modify the ability for transmission of disease. The diseases considered below must be distinguished from disease resulting from contamination of units of blood during the collection process. As these conditions are discussed, we will emphasize the possibility of formulating regulations which exclude the dangerous donor, and the practicality of screening tests will be mentioned.

Although a wide variety of communicable diseases can, in theory, be transmitted by blood transfusion, those conditions of most concern to blood bankers on a world-wide basis are malaria, Chagas' disease, and viral hepatitis. The latter assumes the greatest importance in terms of morbidity and mortality. The problems of the risk, transmission, detection, and prevention of hepatitis have been reviewed thoroughly elsewhere. Therefore, emphasis in the ensuing discussion will be placed on the remainder of diseases transmissable by transfusion. Moreover, we will focus attention on the recent emergence of Cytomegalovirus, Epstein-Barr Virus, and Toxoplasmosis as possible complications of blood transfusion.

Malaria

It has been known for almost a century that malaria can be transmitted by blood inoculation, although the first case of posttransfusion malaria was not reported until 1911. At that time Woolsey described a patient with pernicious anemia who developed Vivax malaria after direct transfusion of blood.[1] The donor denied ever having had the disease. During subsequent years, reports of malaria transmitted by blood transfusion became increasingly common, paralleling the increased use of the procedure. Use of direct transfusion during the third and fourth decades of this century placed the donor, as well as the recipient, at risk of contracting malaria. The incidence of malaria then decreased as more attention was placed on the selection of donors and the preservation of blood.

It has been estimated that approximately 350 cases of accidentally induced malaria, with 250 of these cases resulting from blood transfusion, were reported in the world literature between 1911 and 1950, and that 60% of these cases were due to *P. vivax*.[2] Since 1950 over 1,200 accidentally induced cases have been reported, the majority resulting from blood transfusion, and approximately ⅔ of these were due to *P. malariae*. This reflects the increasing and widespread use of transfusion as a therapeutic tool and the difficulty of excluding the donor with *P. malariae* infection.

This increased world-wide incidence is misleading in assessing the extent of the problem in the United States. Between 1958 and 1971 there were 37 cases reported in this country.[3] During the preceding decade, 12 cases were reported. Therefore, posttransfusion malaria has never been a significant cause of recipient morbidity. Nevertheless, this must be considered in the differential diagnosis of fever of undetermined origin in a patient who has had a recent transfusion of red cell products. Similarly, in the United Kingdom, only six cases of posttransfusion malaria were reported between 1936 and 1970.[2] Much higher incidences have been reported from the Balkans, even from those countries where malaria eradication programs have been successful. The prevalence of *P. malariae* in such areas is related to the fact that quartan malaria may remain as a latent infection for many years.

In the United States most recent cases of posttransfusion malaria have been related to blood donors who had military service in Southeast Asia. It has been estimated that one percent of returning United States troops were infected, with *P. vivax* being the most common parasite. Reported instances of malaria transmission have followed transfusion not only of whole blood and red blood cells, but also of platelet products and leukocyte concentrates, preparations unavoidably contaminated with red blood cells.[4]

Review of the 37 cases reported in the United States during the 1958-1971 interval indicates that rigorous application of the Standards of the AABB would have prevented all but two of the cases. One was a donor with *P. malariae* who had emigrated to the continental United

States from Puerto Rico six years before the blood donation, and the other was a Mexican who had come to the United States 11 years before donation and also transmitted *P. malariae*. Only 3 cases of posttransfusion malaria were reported in the United States in 1972, compared with 8 cases in 1970 and 4 cases in 1971.

In at least 75 percent of the reported cases of posttransfusion malaria, the infection occurred following transfusion of blood stored for less than six days. Only two cases have been reported wherein blood was stored for more than two weeks. It has been demonstrated that all species of Plasmodia may survive at 4 C for many weeks; furthermore, Plasmodia can withstand storage at −79 C for several months.[2]

The longevity of *P. falciparum* in man seldom exceeds one year. *Plasmodium vivax* usually dies out within three years, whereas *P. malariae* may persist for many years in blood.[5] There have been only rare instances of posttransfusion malaria resulting from donors who have had asymptomatic infection approaching three years due either to *P. vivax* or *P. falciparum*. The longevity of *P. ovale* averages 26 months.[3] In contrast, *P. malariae* may persist in the asymptomatic patient for many years. The number of parasites of *P. malariae* in the peripheral blood may be scanty and often is below the threshold of microscopic examination. The frequent inability to detect parasites in the blood of infective donors with *P. malariae* infection, even using special technics, compounds the problem of prevention.[6]

The prevention of posttransfusion malaria centers on two situations: definitions of areas of the world which should be considered endemic, and restrictions which should be applied to potential donors. The Standards of the AABB have never defined endemic areas. Rather, they refer to the World Health Organization list and map, thereby permitting revision of the list as frequently as necessary by knowledgeable consultants.

In terms of donor restrictions, those writing the Standards are concerned not only with prevention of posttransfusion malaria, but also with the danger of reducing the nation's blood supply through excessively restrictive regulations. According to the Center for Disease Control, all reported cases of posttransfusion malaria in the United States in recent years have occurred within three years of the donor's entry into this country, with the exception of the two cases of quartan malaria noted above. Therefore, the three-year waiting interval seems both practical and logical. As recommended by the Center for Disease Control, the donor who has had chemoprophylaxis, and returning servicemen from endemic areas are excluded for three years. This regulation is based on the rarity of recrudescense of malaria beyond three years after discontinuance of treatment and after the potential donor has become asymptomatic.

Finally, the six-month exclusion for the transient visitor to an endemic area, who has not taken chemoprophylaxis, may appear illogical, especially since it takes only an instant for the mosquito to transmit the disease. However, the long-standing application of this guideline indicates it does not present a danger to the recipient population. Moreover, extension of this rule to a three-year exclusion would eliminate a large segment of the blood donor population.

Herpes Virus Infections

The cytomegaloviruses and the recently-described Epstein-Barr virus, members of the Herpes virus group, have been increasingly incriminated in posttransfusion disease. Initial recognition of these infections related to the definition of the postperfusion syndrome, also termed posttransfusion mononucleosis. This syndrome initially was recognized as a late complication of open heart surgery. It is characterized by fever, splenomegaly and atypical lymphocytosis presenting three to five weeks after transfusion in approximately five percent of patients with this procedure. Skin eruptions have been described, as have abnormal liver function tests. Lymphadenopathy and pharyngitis usually are absent and tests for heterophile antibodies almost always are negative. Since its initial recognition, it has been recognized that this syndrome also can appear, although less frequently, after any blood transfusion. Reported cases have in common the administration of fresh blood, often in large volumes. There is now good evidence that this syndrome most frequently is associated with infection by the Epstein-Barr virus or by cytomegaloviruses.

Epstein-Barr Virus

The Epstein-Barr virus (EBV) is a Herpes-like virus which, since 1968, has been causally related to infectious mononucleosis. This virus originally was noted in specimens from children with Burkitt's lymphoma, and subsequently was shown by the Henles and their associates to result in consistent antibody production during and after clinical attacks of infectious mononucleosis.[7] The virus persists in the lymphoreticular system following primary infection and circulates in the blood, probably within leukocytes. As a result, transmission by blood transfusion becomes possible.

Studies of serums for antibody to EBV indicate that infection by the virus is widespread. Moreover, the age of acquisition of the infection can be correlated with socioeconomic conditions. For example, in areas of Africa where Burkitt's lymphoma is prevalent, 90 percent of the children have antibodies to EBV by age 2. Prevalence of 75 percent to 95 percent is found among college students in the Phillipines and Africa, whereas Yale, Smith, and University of Wisconsin undergraduates have prevalence rates varying from 25 percent to 45 percent.[8] Clinical infectious mononucleosis is associated with population groups who have lower prevalence rates of antibody.

In patients with infectious mononucleosis, both heterophile and EBV antibody appear at the time of, or soon after, onset of symptoms. While the heterophile titer declines and disappears relatively quickly, the EBV antibody titer remains at peak levels for several weeks and stabilizes at somewhat lower levels for many years. Tests for EBV antibodies find use in the diagnosis of infectious mononucleosis in patients who do not manifest a heterophile antibody response or who have atypical clinical features. Approximately 10 percent of adults and a greater percentage of children with infectious mononucleosis have negative tests for heterophile antibodies with otherwise typical disease. It must be recognized that illness similar to infectious mononucleosis, lacking a heterophile response, may be produced by cytomegaloviruses, toxoplasma, as well as other viruses.

Gerber, and his associates, noted the relation between EBV and the postperfusion syndrome.[9] Of five patients free of antibody to EBV preoperatively, four had antibody postoperatively, and one of these had clinical infectious mononucleosis. Nevertheless, EBV-associated mononucleosis after perfusion is rare, since most patients have the antibody before the operation.[10] Another study indicated that less than 10 percent of patients undergoing open heart surgery lacked antibody to EBV before operation. In the latter study, eight percent of patients manifested postoperative antibody responses to EBV, but none had signs of illness, supporting the general conclusion that asymptomatic infection is more common than overt illness.

In addition to the postperfusion syndrome, there have been isolated reports of posttransfusion infectious mononucleosis, not only following administration of whole blood, but also after transfusion of platelet-rich plasma.[11] Such cases usually have involved donors who developed infectious mononucleosis within a few days following their donation of blood. The risk of such infection is related to the presence of EBV antibody in the recipient, as well as to the use of freshly drawn blood products.

Cytomegaloviruses

The infectious agents most often causally related to the postperfusion syndrome are the cytomegaloviruses (CMV). This association first was noted in 1966.[12] As is the case with EBV, the vast majority of CMV infections detected after open heart surgery remain silent and are evident only by the subsequent appearance of antibody. The cardiopulmonary bypass plays no role in the production of this syndrome; rather, it is related to the volume and freshness of transfused blood.[13] Although clinically indistinguishable, posttransfusion mononucleosis due to CMV or EBV are etiologically discrete entities. The greater frequency of CMV in these cases is related to the far greater incidence of pre-existing antibodies to EBV before the operation. A recent study indicated that 40 percent of patients lacked antibody to CMV, while only 10 percent lacked antibody to EBV.[10]

The CMV are members of the Herpes virus family.[14] *In vivo* the viruses produce striking cytomegaly with intranuclear inclusion bodies in epithelial cells. The CMV are antigenically heterogenous and by adulthood a majority of persons have serologic evidence of past infection, usually clinically inapparent. CMV and EBV are similar in their capacity to induce chronic infection of circulating lymphocytes. Furthermore, the clinical association of CMV mononucleosis with transfusion of blood less than 48 hours old further indicts the viable white blood cell as the carrier of the virus.

Primary infection with CMV may be acquired prenatally as a result of transplacental passage or through intrauterine transfusion,[15] perinatally from infected cervical secretions, or postnatally. The latter infections may be acquired from blood transfusion, organ transplantation, or from contact with infected secretions or excretions. Furthermore, there may be reinfection from similar sources with reactivation of latent infection in the patient. The latter process is especially important in patients with debilitating disease or in patients receiving immunosuppressive therapy.

Prenatal involvement by CMV may produce disease ranging from severe brain damage and deafness to virtually asymptomatic infection. In contrast, infection in children and adults usually spares the nervous system. The syndrome termed "CMV mononucleosis" is identical hematologically with infectious mononucleosis; however, it lacks significant pharyngeal involvement, lymphadenopathy and heterophile antibodies. Hemolytic anemia and thrombocytopenia are common in congenital infections, and the former must be differentiated from hemolytic disease of the newborn due to blood group antibodies.

Clinical CMV infection in blood recipients may be manifested by the mononucleosis-like syndrome or by an interstitial pneumonitis, the latter occurring predominantly in patients on immunosuppressive therapy. It is debatable whether these posttransfusion complications represent endogenous or exogenous infection, although both may occur. Nevertheless, the three to five week latent interval for postperfusion syndrome and the production of IgM antibody to CMV in many such patients strongly supports the concept of primary infection.

Although a protective effect of pre-existing antibody has been reported by some authors, it has not been observed by others.[16] This may be related to the serologic heterogeneity of different strains of CMV. Moreover, transfused virus may not be readily neutralized due to the intracellular location of the virus.

It is not feasible to exclude as donors of blood those with demonstrable antibody either to CMV or EBV. This would eliminate the majority of potential blood donors. Moreover, viremia in such donors is likely to be intermittent, and recipients with serologic evidence of prior infection may be resistant. A more logical course may be to avoid indiscriminate administration of blood less than 48 hours old when possible. Although antibody evidence of infection may occur when older blood is transfused, clinically manifest infections are uncommon.

Toxoplasmosis

There have been several reports of posttransfusion toxoplasmosis, all in recipients of white blood cell transfusions collected from donors with chronic myelogenous leukemia.[17, 18] The recipients in each instance, because of their basic disease process, as well as immunosuppressive therapy, were unusually susceptible to infection with this organism.

Toxoplasmosis results from infection with *Toxoplasma gondii,* a unique microorganism.[19] Generally classified as a protozoan, it is an obligate intracellular parasite capable of living and multiplying in virtually all cells except non-nucleated red blood cells. It also has the ability to encyst and remain alive in a host virtually indefinitely. It survives in citrated blood for at least 50 days at 4 C.[20] Through parasitemia the organism can become widely disseminated. While the finding of organisms indicates infection, it does not necessarily indicate disease. For example, in the United States, depending upon locale studied, between 5 and 60 percent of the population manifests antibody. Nonetheless, evidence of clinical disease is meager in all such areas.

Transmission of toxoplasmosis may be by several routes, including ingestion of infected meat, transplacentally from mother to fetus, and through contact with cat excreta. *Toxocara catis,* a nematode which parasitizes cats, may become infected when the cat eats infected mice. The Toxocara eggs, thereby infected, are then excreted by the cat.

Although clinical manifestations are uncommon in the mother, the baby with congenital toxoplasmosis may have a characteristic tetrad of chorioretinitis, hydrocephalus or microcephalus, psychomotor retardation, and cerebral calcification.

Acquired toxoplasmosis usually is asymptomatic, or is an unrecognized innocuous infection. It may be characterized by low grade fever, variable skin eruption, lymph node enlargement, and lymphocytosis. Rarely myocarditis, encephalitis, or pneumonitis may occur.

Immunologically compromised patients may develop disseminated toxoplasmosis. Such infection has been transmitted to these patients not only by transfusion, but also by organ transplantation. Presumably the cysts rupture, releasing free trophozoytes which are responsible for dissemination.

The high proportion of positive tests for antibody to toxoplasmosis using the Sabin-Feldman dye test mitigates the value of this test for detection of infection. Cases transmitted by leukocyte transfusion likely result from use of blood with large numbers of parasitized cells. Miller, et al, isolated *T. gondii* from the buffy coat of patients with myelogenous leukemia.[21] Proof of primary infection in the recipient rests on negative antibody titers before transfusion and elevated titers during the acute illness.

It has been suggested that persons with significantly elevated titers of antibodies to toxoplasmosis be rejected as donors of white blood cells to unusually susceptible patients.[17] However, donor parasitemia is the critical factor, and is extremely rare in well donors. This would explain the donor-patient findings in the reported cases and the paucity of reports with other forms of transfusion.

Syphilis

The transmission of syphilis by blood transfusion first was documented in 1915. Subsequent reports of such transmission uniformly implicated donors with primary or secondary lues. Several instances of transmission from asymptomatic seronegative donors have been reported.[22] The latter readily can be explained by noting the relationship of seropositivity and spirochaetemia to the various stages of the disease.

Treponema pallidum does not survive more than 72 hours in citrated blood.[23] Therefore, the danger of transmission of syphilis exists primarily with fresh blood transfusion. This is illustrated by the patient reported by Chambers, et al, who developed the rash of secondary lues following transfusion of platelet concentrates.[24] *Treponema pallidum* may remain viable when stored for extended periods at –45 C, or below, although it is killed by lyophilization.

The administration of blood with a positive serologic test for syphilis (STS) will convert the recipient to seropositivity. Walker stored 98 units of STS positive blood for seven days and then transfused them to 90 patients. The resulting positive STS in the recipients disappeared in four to ten days.[25]

Although neither the transmission of the disease, nor the transmission of seropositivity assumes great clinical significance, it must be noted that a positive STS may be due to a wide variety of conditions other than syphilis. Most of these conditions would exclude a potential blood donor. Therefore, it would seem prudent to exclude all prospective donors with a consistently positive STS which cannot be otherwise explained.

Trypanosomiasis and Leishmaniasis

Reports of transmission of African trypanosomiasis and Kala Azar by blood transfusion are exceedingly rare.[26,27] However, posttransfusion Chagas' disease is a major public health problem in endemic areas. Infection with *Trypanosoma cruzi*, the etiologic agent of Chagas' disease, assumes considerable importance in areas of South and Central America. In some parts of Latin America as many as 50 percent of potential blood donors are infected. It is estimated that over seven million people in the "Chagas belt," between Northern Argentina and Southern Mexico, are infected with *T. cruzi*. The vast majority of these individuals have asymptomatic disease.

Chagas' disease usually is a mild infection, manifested by edema, fever, and lymphadenopathy, symptoms which may simulate the patient's primary disease.[28] While the acute infection has a mortality rate of five to ten percent, at least an additional ten percent of patients develop cardiac involvement which ultimately may lead to death.

The usual mode of transmission of Chagas' disease in Latin America is through the bite of the infected reduviid bug. However, in many areas blood transfusion is the second most important means of transmitting this condition. *T. cruzi* maintains some infective capacity when blood is stored at 4 C for 21 days; however, blood stored beyond ten days rarely produces infection.

The problem of this infection is of sufficient magnitude in endemic areas that it has been proposed to incorporate crystal violet in the anticoagulant solution for blood preservation.[28] A complement-fixation test is used widely in South America to detect latent disease, and has been used for exclusion of donors.

OTHER DISEASES TRANSMISSIBLE BY BLOOD TRANSFUSION

Brucellosis

Only one well-documented case of brucellosis has been reported following blood transfusion.[29] In that report the recipient developed symptoms and signs of brucellosis 13 weeks following transfusion. The patient manifested malaise, anorexia, fever, myalgia, hepatosplenomegaly, and his serum agglutinated *B. abortus* at 1:2560. Two other incompletely documented cases have been reported from Mexico.

Although the causative organisms for brucellosis remain viable at 4 C for months, the number of organisms in the prodromal patient's blood is usually scanty. Furthermore, they would be destroyed by most recipients. This likely is the explanation for the rarity of this complication.

Typhus

Only one case of posttransfusion typhus has been reported.[30] The donor, in this report from Germany during World War II, developed clinical disease two days after blood donation, whereas the recipient manifested symptoms 11 days later.

Filariasis

Transfusion of blood with microfilaria will not produce filariasis in the recipient, since the mosquito vector is essential for development of the organism. This explains why filariasis has not followed deliberate transfusion of blood containing microfilaria, although transient allergic manifestations may occur.

The presence of these organisms in donor blood may make for an alarming observation during pretransfusion testing and may cause concern for the blood bank technologist. The vigorous motility of microfilaria can be seen with the naked eye. It should be appreciated that microfilaria of *W. bancrofti, L. loa,* and *D. perstans* may remain viable in stored donor blood for at least two weeks.[31]

Measles

In spite of the prevalence of measles in this country, there has been only a single report of its transmission by blood transfusion.[32] Two infants who developed the disease after receiving direct transfusions from their mothers were documented in that paper. The mothers were well at the time of the transfusion, but developed measles within the following two days, whereas the infants had a two-week incubation period.

Salmonellosis

To exemplify the fact that any organism in the blood of a donor may produce disease in a recipient, transmission of *Salmonella cholerasuis* was reported in seven patients who received platelets donated by a single individual. In this report, the donor had concealed the presence of chronic osteomyelitis due to the organism in question and the infected recipients of the platelet transfusions were immunologically compromised through chemotherapy.

Colorado Tick Fever

This is a flu-like illness, usually self-limited, and characterized by fever, chills, headache, and nausea and vomiting. The disease is prevalent in the western United States and it is transmitted by the wood tick, *D. andersoni.* The virus has been demonstrated in plasma during the acute illness and in the patient's red blood cells for up to three months after infection. Furthermore, the disease has been transmitted by accidental innoculation by needles contaminated with the virus. However, at this time there is no firm evidence of transmission of this disease by blood transfusion.

REFERENCES

1. Woolsey G: Transfusion for pernicious anemia: two cases. *Ann. Surg.* **53**:132, 1911.
2. Chwatt LJB: Blood transfusion and tropical disease. *Trop. Dis. Bull* **69**:825, 1972.
3. Dover AS, Schultz MG: Transfusion-induced malaria. *Transfusion* **11**:353, 1971.
4. Dover AS, Guinee VF: Malaria transmission by leukocyte component therapy. *J.A.M.A.* **217**:1701, 1971.
5. Parasitology of Malaria: World Health Organization Technical Report Series, No. 433. Geneva, World Health Organization, 1969, p. 29.
6. Grant DB, Permpanayagam MS, Shute P, et al: A case of malignant tertian malaria after blood transfusion. *Lancet* **2**:469, 1970.
7. Henle G, Henle W, Diehl V: Relation of Burkitt's tumor-associated herpes-type virus to infectious mononucleosis. *Proc. Natl. Acad. Sci. USA* **59**:94, 1968.
8. Henle G, Henle W: EB virus in the etiology of infectious mononucleosis. *Hosp. Practice* **5**:33, 1970.
9. Gerber P, Walsh JH, Rosenblum EN, et al: Association of EB virus infection with the postperfusion syndrome. *Lancet* **1**:593, 1969.
10. Henle W, Henle G, Scriba M, et al: Antibody responses to the Epstein-Barr virus and cytomegaloviruses after open-heart and other surgery. *N. Engl. J. Med.* **282**:1068, 1970.
11. Turner A: Transmission of infectious mononucleosis by transfusion of pre-illness plasma. *Ann. Int. Med.* **77**:751, 1972.
12. Kaariainen L, Klemola E, Poloheimo J: Rise of cytomegalovirus antibodies in an infectious mononucleosis-like syndrome after transfusion. *Br. Med. J.* **1**:1270, 1966.
13. Stevens D, Barker LF, Ketcham AS, et al: Asymptomatic cytomegalovirus infection following blood transfusion in tumor surgery. *J.A.M.A.* **211**:1341, 1970.
14. Weller TH: The cytomegaloviruses: ubiquitous agents with protean clinical manifestations. *N. Engl. J. Med.* **285**:203, 267, 1971.

15. King-Lewis PA, Gardner SD: Congenital cytomegalic inclusion disease following intrauterine transfusion. *Br. Med. J.* **1**:603, 1969.

16. Prince AM, Szmuness W, Millian SJ, et al: A serologic study of cytomegalovirus infections associated with blood transfusions. *N. Engl. J. Med.* **284**:1125, 1971.

17. Roth JA, Siegel SE, Levine A, et al: Fatal recurrent toxoplasmosis in a patient initially infected via a leukocyte transfusion. *Am. J. Clin. Pathol.* **56**:601, 1971.

18. Siegel SE, Lunde MN, Gelderman AH: Transmission of toxoplasmosis by leukocyte transfusion. *Blood* **37**:388, 1971.

19. Feldman HA: Toxoplasma and toxoplasmosis. *Hosp. Practice* **4**:64, 1969.

20. Kimball AC, Kean BH, Kellner A: The risk of transmitting toxoplasmosis by blood transfusion. *Transfusion* **5**:447, 1965.

21. Miller MJ, Aronson W, Remington JS: Late parasitemia in asymptomatic acquired toxoplasmosis. *Ann. Int. Med.* **71**:139, 1967.

22. McCluskie JA: The transmission of syphilis by blood transfusion. *Br. Med. J.* **1**:264, 1939.

23. Bloch O: Loss of virulence of *Treponema pallidum* in citrated blood at 5 C. *Bull. J. Hopkins Hosp.* **68**:412, 1941.

24. Chambers RW, Foley HT, Schmidt PJ: Transmission of syphilis by fresh blood components. *Transfusion.* **9**:32, 1969.

25. Walker RH: The disposition of STS-reactive blood in a transfusion service. *Transfusion* **5**:452, 1965.

26. Ferreira FS, Rosano JM: A case of human trypanosomiasis transmitted by blood transfusion. *Graz. Med. Portug.* **4**:1030, 1951.

27. Chung H, Chou H, Lu J: The first two cases of transfusion kala azar. *Chinese Med. J. (Shanghai)* **66**:325, 1948.

28. Rivero I: Chagas disease— another hazard in acute leukemia. *N. Engl. J. Med.* **290**:285, 1974.

29. Vilaseia GC, Cerisola JA, Olarte JA, et al: The use of crystal violet in the prevention of the transfusional transmission of Chagas-Mazza disease. *Vox Sang.* **11**:711, 1966.

30. Wood E: Brucellosis as a hazard of blood transfusion. *Br. Med. J.* **1**:27, 1955.

31. Dormanns E, Emminger E: Transmission of typhus fever from man to man by blood transfusion in the incubation period. *Munch. Med. Wochenschr.* **89**:559, 1942.

32. Bird G, Menon K: Survival of *Microfilaria bancrofti* in stored blood. *Lancet* **2:**721, 1961.
33. Bauguess H: Measles transmitted by blood transfusion. *Am. J. Dis. Child.* **27**:256, 1924.
34. Rhame FS, Root RK, MacLowry JD, et al: Salmonella septicemia from platelet transfusions. *Ann. Int. Med.* **78**:633, 1973.
35. Philip RN: Can blood transfusions spread tick fever? *J.A.M.A.* **225**:575, 1973.

PREPARATION AND STORAGE OF PLATELET CONCENTRATES

Sherrill J. Slichter
and
Laurence A. Harker

Introduction

AN ADEQUATE supply of platelets is more difficult to provide than red cells because the platelets harvested from several units of whole blood are needed for an effective dose. The increasing use of platelet transfusions, as well as the dose required, necessitates improved efficiency in blood bank operation to meet the needs for platelets as well as other blood components. Administration of platelets as concentrates rather than as whole blood not only makes it possible to give patients the number of platelets they need, but also promotes improvement in blood utilization, since the remaining plasma and red cells can be used for other purposes. For effective blood bank operation and patient care, concentrates should contain the maximum number of viable, functional platelets. In addition, the need for platelets in emergency situations requires the use of efficient storage techniques. In our laboratory we have investigated each step in the preparation and storage of platelets by measuring the effect of various conditions on platelet yield in the concentrate as well as subsequent viability and function. After completion of studies in normal subjects, fresh and stored concentrates were transfused into aplastic, thrombocytopenic, nonimmunized patients with platelet counts less than $10,000/\mu l$ and bleeding times greater than 60 minutes. Platelet survival was evaluated by measuring ^{51}Cr radioactivity[4] and platelet counts, while function was assessed from the template bleeding time.[5]

The results obtained from these studies indicated the best methods for preparing and storing platelet concentrates for periods up to three days. These techniques are briefly outlined in the following paragraphs.

Preparation of Platelet Concentrates for Storage

A. *Collection*

1. Skin cleansing

The only time the plastic bag system is entered during preparation and storage is during the initial phlebotomy. It is very important to maintain strict asepsis, treating the site of venipuncture as if it were to undergo surgery. This step is much more critical when drawing blood to be used for platelet harvesting than for other uses as platelet concentrates are stored at room temperature.

   2. Plastic bag

A Fenwal double or triple bag containing CPD anticoagulant with transfer packs made of PL-146 plastic should be used (GF-25 or GF-35). A total of 450 cc of blood is collected into the 63 grams of CPD.

   3. Drawing

Standard practices for blood collection with particular emphasis on aseptic techniques provide platelets suitable for storage.

B. *Processing*

   1. Temperature

The blood should be maintained at room temperature (22 C ± 2) until preparation of the platelet concentrate (PC) as refrigeration impairs platelet resuspension and viability. Platelet harvesting must be completed within 6 hours of blood drawing since Factor VIII levels in the residual platelet-poor plasma (PPP) decrease after longer intervals, reducing Factor VIII yield in cryoprecipitates.

   2. Centrifugation

It is possible to recover 89% of the platelets into the platelet-rich plasma (PRP) by spinning the whole blood (WB) for 9 minutes at a g force of 1000 (1900 RPM) in a Sorvall RC-3 swinging bucket horizontal head centrifuge thermostatically controlled at room temperature. After transfer of the PRP to a satellite bag, a g force of 3000 (3300 RPM) for 20 minutes concentrates the platelets into a button containing 86% of the platelets originally present in the WB. To achieve these results it is critical that the machine time and force of centrifugation be accurately calibrated and that the braking time adds no more than two minutes to the centrifugation time. The older procedures for platelet concentrate preparation[1] specify an initial centrifugation of 4470 × g for 3 minutes followed by a hard spin at 5000 × g for 5 minutes, which permits a platelet yield of approximately 41%; i.e., about half the amount obtainable by the method just outlined.

   3. Resuspension

After a 1 to 2 hour undisturbed rest at room temperature, the platelets are resuspended by gentle manual manipulation[9] into 50 to 60 cc of residual plasma. The appropriate amount of plasma can be approximated by placing two pennies in the upper corners of a plasma expressor and clamping off the connecting tubing when the movable plate meets the pennies. The excess platelet-poor plasma is either returned to the red cells or transferred to a second satellite bag for preparation of fresh frozen plasma or cryoprecipitate. If the platelets are not resuspended gently, irreversible clumping occurs, reducing the number of platelets which circulate as the aggregates are either trapped in the blood filter or removed by the spleen. If the platelets start to aggregate during manipulation, a further waiting period is required.

Storage Requirements

A. *Preparation of the platelet concentrate*

The concentrate should be prepared as outlined above. Although higher centrifugation forces than $3000 \times g$ for 20 minutes; i.e., $4000 \times g$ for 10 minutes, reduces the preparation time while still concentrating all the platelets into a button, this g force is associated with significant decreases in posttransfusion platelet viability after 72 hours of storage.

B. *Temperature*

Platelet recovery (the percentage of transfused platelets which circulate immediately posttransfusion) after 24 to 72 hours of storage is comparable for both 22 and 4 C temperature, but the platelets stored at the former temperature have an average survival of eight days in contrast to one day for the latter, as previously reported.[2, 8, 10] There are also differences in function. The 4 C stored platelets only shorten the bleeding time of half the patients receiving these transfusions, and in those who do show some benefit, the duration is only about 4 hours. Conversely, 22 C stored platelets are comparable to fresh platelets, shortening the bleeding time to an extent appropriate for the number of circulating platelets. If the platelet donors have been taking aspirin, the transfused platelets are dysfunctional although functional integrity returns "in vivo" 4 to 8 hours posttransfusion. This delayed improvement of the bleeding time with donors who have been on aspirin is more commonly found after transfusing room temperature stored platelets rather than fresh.

C. *Anticoagulant*

After 24 hours of storage, platelet recovery is comparable for ACD and CPD, but after 72 hours, the CPD stored platelet recovery is 12% better than that of those stored in ACD.

D. *Plasma resuspending volume*

When platelets are to be stored more than 24 hours; an increase in the volume of residual plasma from 20cc to 60cc is required to prevent an undesirable drop in pH. There is a direct inverse relationship between increasing platelet count and decreasing pH during storage. When the pH is 6.3 to 6.4 there is minimal loss of viability; at pH 6 or below, the platelets are almost totally nonviable. The fact that CPD has a higher initial pH (7.2) compared to ACD (7.0) may account for the better results with this anticoagulant.

E. *Storage bag*

The plastic composition of the transfer bag affects platelet viability even after 24 hours of storage. Platelets stored in Fenwal's PL-146 bag had normal recoveries and survivals; those stored in McGaw (Double Hemo-Pak, T2205, ACD-A) showed an average reduction in recovery of 3%, and survival shortened by a half-day; with Cutter bags (PR 2370A, ACD-A) there was a 34% decrease in recovery and a one day loss of survival. After 72 hours of storage, Fenwal's PL-146 and McGaw bags showed the same relative differences in platelet viability.

F. *Mixing*

Without constant gentle mixing to prevent the platelets from settling, platelet recovery after 24 hours of storage is only half of that obtained with mixing, and survival is decreased by 1.5 days. A circular rotator platform is used in our laboratory, and the platelet bags are placed individually on open wire racks with fans at both ends to circulate the air and prevent the heat of the motors from increasing the temperature. Recent studies suggest that there is an exchange of oxygen and carbon dioxide between the contents of the bag and the surrounding air, which may contribute to maintaining platelet viability during storage.[11] This type of open storage arrangement which increases the contact between bags and the surrounding air may be important.

Quality of the Product

A comprehensive platelet transfusion program must include a system to monitor the yield of platelets in the concentrates after preparation and the viability and function of the platelets after storage, as well as their sterility.

A. *Platelet yield*

Percent platelet yield is calculated by:
$$\frac{\text{platelet count of concentrate} \times \text{concentrate volume}}{\text{donor's platelet count} \times \text{volume of blood collected}} \times 100.$$ This should average 86%. Reduced platelet yields are usually due to improper standardization of centrifuge timing or RPM's or prolonged braking intervals. Alternate explanations are failure to transfer all the platelet-rich plasma from the residual red cells (280cc ± 10) into the transfer pack or faulty resuspension, so that platelet aggregates are formed, and several platelets are counted as one.

B. *Viability*

1. *In vitro*

Routine monitoring of the pH of platelet concentrates after 72 hours of storage identifies nonviable units with a pH of less than 6.0. Inadequate amounts of residual plasma usually accounts for this problem. However, storage temperatures above 24 C (a thermometer should be placed in the storage area), inadequate mixing, so that cells are collected in the bottom of the bag, or decreased air-bag interfaces also cause a fall in pH and associated loss of viability.

2. *In vivo*

Pre- and posttransfusion platelet counts should be determined when pooled fresh and stored platelet concentrates are administered to *appropriate* aplastic, thrombocytopenic recipients; i.e., exclude patients with disease-associated platelet destruction (allo- or autoantibodies, viremia, or conditions associated with intravascular hemostatic factor consumption;[6] i.e., disseminated malignancies, septicemias, or tissue injury). In properly chosen patients, we have found the average recovery of both fresh and room temperature stored platelets to be approximately 38% and survival five days. Aplastic, thrombocytopenic patients consistently have modest reductions in platelet survivals so the normal range in these patients is four to six days.

C. *Function*

Pre- and posttransfusion bleeding times should be correlated with platelet counts for at least 24 hours. With proper platelet function, the bleeding time is predicted by the following equation:

bleeding time (minutes) $= 30.5 - (\frac{\text{platelet count}/\mu l}{3,850})$ when the platelet count is between 20,000 and 100,000/μl. It is important, if possible, that each patient serve as his own control so that disease or drug associated platelet dysfunction which would prolong the bleeding time does not suggest dysfunction of the stored platelets.

D. *Bacteriologic monitoring*

The platelet concentrates stored for 72 hours are sampled and inoculated into at least thioglycolate culture medium, which is incubated at both 22 and 37 C. Although platelet contamination with subsequent growth of organisms during room temperature storage is of major concern, actual data suggest that this rarely occurs[3,7] and even that platelet concentrates have some bacteriocidal capacity.[12] If contaminated cultures are identified, the method of cleansing the donor's skin before the venipuncture should be examined, and the plastic storage bags should be searched for leaks.

Summary

A technique of platelet storage is presented which permits the maximum number of viable and functional platelets to be preserved for periods of 72 hours without bacterial contamination. The requirements must be followed rigidly, but the method is simple to perform and does not require expensive equipment. Important factors include: (1) preparation from whole blood drawn after thorough skin cleansing, (2) blood collection into CPD, (3) centrifugation of the PRP at low g forces (3000 $\times$ g for 20 minutes), (4) 60cc residual plasma volume, (5) a storage bag composed of Fenwal's PL-146 plastic, (6) room temperature 22 C $\pm$ 2, and (7) constant gentle agitation during storage. Platelet viability after 72 hours of storage as measured by *in vivo* recovery and survival shows an 8% decrease in the former compared to fresh platelets (54 to 46%) and a 0.5 day shortening of the latter (8.4 to 7.9 days). The function of these platelets as measured by the correlation between bleeding time and platelet count after transfusion of pooled platelets into aplastic, thrombocytopenic recipients shows as good or better function when compared to fresh platelets.

REFERENCES

1. American Association of Blood Banks: *Technical Methods and Procedures,* ed. 5, p 169, 1970.
2. Becker GA, Tuccelli M, Kunicki T, Chalos MK, Aster RH: Studies of Platelet Concentrates Stored at 22 C and 4 C. *Transfusion* **13**:61, 1973.
3. Goddard D, Jacobs SI, Manohitharajah SM: The Bacteriological Screening of Platelet Concentrates Stored at 22 C. *Transfusion* **13**:103, 1973.
4. Harker LA, Finch CA: Thrombokinetics in Man. *J Clin Invest* **48**:963, 1969.
5. Harker LA, Slichter SJ: The Bleeding Time as a Screening Test for Evaluation of Platelet Function. *New Engl J Med* **287**:155, 1972.
6. Harker LA, Slichter SJ: Platelet and Fibrinogen Consumption in Man. *New Engl J Med* **287**:999, 1972.
7. Katz A, Tilton R: Sterility of Platelet Concentrates Stored at 25 C. Transfusion **10**:329, 1970.
8. Levin R, Freireich E: Effect of Storage up to 48 hours on Response to Transfusion of Platelet-Rich Plasma. *Transfusion* **4**:251, 1964.
9. Mourad N: A Simple Method for Obtaining Platelet Concentrates Free of Aggregates. *Transfusion* **8**:48, 1968.
10. Murphy S, Gardner F: Platelet Preservation. Effect of Storage Temperature on Maintenance of Platelet Viability—Deleterious Effect of Refrigerated Storage. *New Engl J Med* **280**:1094, 1969.
11. Murphy S, Gardner FH: The Role of Plastic Type and the Pasteur Effect in the Storage of Platelets for Transfusion at 22 C. *26th Annual AABB Program Manual,* abstract p. 101, 1973.
12. Myhre BA, Walker LJ, White ML: Bacteriocidal properties of Platelet Concentrates. *Transfusion* **14**:116, 1974.

GRANULOCYTE TRANSFUSION

Jeffrey McCullough

I. Introduction

IN THE late 1950's, the major cause of death in patients with bone marrow failure due to leukemia or aplastic anemia was hemorrhage, with infection a distant second. However, during the last ten years, as the use of platelet transfusions has become commonplace, there has been a dramatic decrease in the incidence of hemorrhage as cause of death in these patients.[16] During the 1965 to 1971 time period, infection accounted for 69% of the deaths in patients with hematologic-malignancy while hemorrhage accounted for only 11% of the deaths in these patients.[23] Thus, with the increasingly aggressive use of chemotherapy and irradiation therapy in patients with malignant diseases, it is crucial that methods be developed to provide treatment of infectious complications which develop during temporary periods of bone marrow suppression. Until recently, granulocyte transfusion has been hampered by difficulty in collecting sufficient numbers of cells to make transfusion practical, and also by an inability to store granulocytes for more than a few hours after collection.

One of the first considerations in granulocyte transfusion is the relationship between the circulating granulocyte level and the risk of infection. Bodey, et al[1] showed that in patients with acute leukemia, 53% of the hospital days were spent with identified infection if the patient's absolute granulocyte count was less than 100 per cubic millimeter. As the absolute granulocyte count increased, the percentage of hospital days spent with infection sharply decreased and reached its minimum when the absolute granulocyte count was greater than 1500 per cubic millimeter. The frequency of episodes of severe infection also was inversely related to the absolute granulocyte count. Thus, it appears that a critical level of circulating granulocytes is 1500 per cubic millimeter. When the absolute granulocyte count falls below this level, the patient's risk of infection begins to increase and the risk and severity of infection continue to increase, the lower the absolute count. These granulocyte levels apply to uninfected patients. It is much more difficult to assess the required granulocyte level which will enable a patient to effectively combat existing infection. In addition, granulocytes must be functional in order to provide the antibacterial activity expected for a given level of circulating granulocytes.

II. Granulocyte collection

Because of the small number of leukocytes in whole blood, compared with red cells and platelets, it has not been practical to collect granulocytes from normal donors by ordinary phlebotomy. In the initial investigation of leukocyte transfusion, granulocytes were obtained by performing leukapheresis on patients with chronic myelogenous leukemia (CML) who had high peripheral granulocyte counts.[9,35,36] However, granulocyte collection from donors with CML is unsatisfactory because of the limited number of donors available, and because of the presence of blasts in the granulocyte concentrate obtained from these patients.

Recently, several methods have been developed for collecting a large number of granulocytes from normal donors. The continuous flow centrifuge (CFC)* was developed jointly by the National Institutes of Health and the IBM Corporation. In this instrument, whole blood flows from the donor into a closed continuous flow system through a centrifuge bowl where it is separated into plasma, buffy coat, and red cells. The buffy coat is removed and collected into a plastic bag while the packed red cells and leukocyte-poor plasma are recombined and returned to the donor via a second venipuncture. The efficiency of leukocyte removal is approximately 25% of the granulocytes which pass through the instrument, so that large volumes of blood must be processed in order to obtain sufficient numbers of cells from normal donors. The donor is anticoagulated either with ACD solution alone or a combination of ACD and heparin. Blood flow rates through the instrument are maintained at approximately 40 ml/min., so that during a typical CFC leukapheresis, approximately 7-10 liters of whole blood are processed and the donor receives 400-500 ml of ACD and 4000-6000 units of heparin.[28] Some investigators utilize large doses of heparin and others use no heparin, but almost twice as much ACD solution.

Using CFC leukapheresis, between .2 and $.79 \times 10^{10}$ granulocytes can be collected from unstimulated normal donors (Table 1). In an effort to obtain larger numbers of granulocytes from normal donors, stimulation of the peripheral granulocyte count with conventional steroids, etiocholanolone and the use of hydroxyethyl starch (HES) to improve the granulocyte separation within the CFC, have been at-

---

* Blood Cell Separator, IBM Corporation, Endicott, N.Y.; Celltrifuge, American Instrument Co., Silver Spring, Md.

TABLE 1: Granulocyte Collection by CFC Leukapheresis of Normal Donors

Unstimulated	Blood Volume Processed (liters)	Time (hrs)	Total WBC's x 10^{10}	Total PMN's x 10^{10}	Reference
M.D. Anderson	10.0	—	1.2	0.2	25
Hospital & Tumor Institute	9.2	—	1.4	0.42	24
National Cancer	—	—	1.1	0.56	11
Institute	8.4	4	1.13	0.49	14
Roswell Park Memorial Institute	—	3-4	1.42	0.79	22
University of Minnesota	7.9	3	0.95	0.47	32
Rochester Regional Red Cross	10.0	—	—	0.4	37
Baltimore Cancer Research Center	—	3.3	—	0.57	2
Steroid Stimulation					
M.D. Anderson	10.0	—	1.9	0.8	25
(etiocholanolone)	9.0	—	1.6	.64	24
Rochester (prednisone)	10.0	—	—	1.0	37
Roswell Park (dexamethasone)	—	3-4	1.5	1.21	22
HES Utilization					
M.D. Anderson	10.0	—	1.8	1.0	25
University of Minnesota	7.9	—	1.51	0.97	32
Steroids and HES					
M.D. Anderson	10.0	—	3.0	2.2	25

tempted.[2,22,24,25,32,37] These methods result in increased granulocyte yields (Table 1); however, such stimulation increases the risk to the donor. The side effects of etiocholanolone include fever and pain at the site of injection. The use of steroids, particularly if donors are to be leukapheresed daily for one to two-week periods, may result in adrenal suppression with possible Addisonian crisis. There exists the possibility of anaphylactic reactions to hydroxyethel starch, although none have been reported.[32] In addition, hydroxyethyl starch is a very potent volume expander, so that headache and possible fluid overload problems may develop as a complication of its prolonged or vigorous use.

In 1966, Greenwalt reported the use of granulocyte adhesion to nylon fibers as a method of preparing leukocyte-poor blood. In 1971, Djerassi[5] described a procedure to reverse the adhesion of granulocytes to nylon fibers, thus making it possible to trap granulocytes selectively on the nylon fibers and prepare a granulocyte concentrate by eluting the cells. The median number of granulocytes collected by this filtration leukapheresis (FL) technique ranges from $1.2 - 4.3 \times 10^{10}$ (Table 2), depending upon the volume of blood processed and the

TABLE 2: Granulocyte Collection by Filtration Leukapheresis of Normal Donors

	Blood Volume Processed	Time	Total WBC's $\times 10^{10}$	Total Granulocytes $\times 10^{10}$	Reference
Mercy Catholic Medical Center, Phila., Pa.	7.2 8.4 9.5	2½ hrs.	3.4 4.0 4.4	3.2 3.8 4.3	6
National Cancer Institute	7.1	2½ hrs.		1.2 2.04	17 15
Baltimore Cancer Research Center		2.3 hrs.		2.1 3.75	2 3
University of Minnesota	11.1	2½ hrs.	1.5	1.4	Unpublished

techniques used. The efficiency of granulocyte collection by FL is much higher than with CFC leukapheresis[15] since most of the granulocytes which pass through the filters adhere to the nylon fibers. In general, it is possible to obtain a larger number of granulocytes in a shorter period of time by FL compared with CFC (Tables 1 and 2). The only anticoagulant used in FL is heparin, since the adherence of granulocytes to the nylon fibers is calcium dependent. Thus, no calcium binding anticoagulant, such as ACD, can be used in the system. Donor reactions do not appear to be more common with FL than CFC leukapheresis; however, extensive data concerning the effects of FL on donors has not yet been published.

Huestis[21] has collected 1.4×10^{10} granulocytes during a 2½ hour leukapheresis using the Haemonetics Model 10 Blood Processor, and we have duplicated these collections in a few donors. The procedure involves the use of ACD anticoagulant and HES. No detailed evaluation of this procedure, or its effects on donors, has appeared in the literature as of this writing.

III. Evaluation of donors prior to leukapheresis and selection of suitable donors.

Because of the extensive manipulation of the donor involved, neither CFC or FL leukapheresis should be undertaken without the careful supervision of a physician. Special attention must be paid to the evaluation of the donor prior to leukapheresis.[28] Potential donors should be subjected to a thorough medical history with special emphasis on questions concerning unusual bleeding, hemoptysis, hematuria, or melena. The donor's veins should be examined for suitability for puncture with a large bore needle. Donors with small or fragile veins should be excluded since the small granulocyte yield from slow blood flow rates will be unsatisfactory. Laboratory testing should include hemoglobin or hematocrit, total leukocyte count and differential, platelet count, and partial thromboplastin time or thrombin time if heparin is used. If ACD anticoagulant is used, determination of serum calcium prior to CFC leukapheresis is optional. In addition, both red cell and white cell compatibility testing must be performed. All these laboratory procedures except the serum calcium can be obtained rather quickly so that it is possible to evaluate the donor in the morning and perform leukapheresis in the afternoon. It is preferable to evaluate the donor further in advance so that histocompatibility testing can be performed and the donor selected accordingly.

The initial hemoglobin should be at least 11 gm/100 ml for a donor to qualify for leukapheresis. If donors are leukapheresed several times weekly, we routinely administer oral iron and vitamin B_{12}. Although we have leukapheresed patients with hemoglobins as low as 8 gm%, most normal donors do not tolerate a hemoglobin value below 9.0 gm%. Transfusions of packed red blood cells to normal related donors are not recommended unless the circumstances are extremely unique. Instead, a different donor should be utilized.

Donors should have a normal platelet count prior to leukapheresis and no leukapheresis procedure should be initiated with a platelet count of less than 125,000/m³. Any abnormality in the coagulation screening should disqualify a potential donor.

We do not feel that a physical examination is required if the medical history is carefully and thoroughly performed. Unusual findings raised by the history should be evaluated by a physician.

Donors undergoing repeated leukapheresis should have a hemoglobin or hematocrit and coagulation tests performed before each leukapheresis. A platelet count should be performed with each donation. Because of the time delay in obtaining the platelet count, we decide on donor suitability based on the platelet count at the termination of the previous procedure.

Selection of the best donor is based on many factors including medical history, laboratory studies, veins, ABO group, and HL-A type, and the donor's personality and motivation.

A granulocyte concentrate contains about 1 gm of hemoglobin so that the red cell group of the donor must be considered. It appears that ABO antigens are on granulocytes[33] and thus even a pure granulocyte suspension would be expected to have a shortened posttransfusion survival in an ABO incompatible recipient. This was confirmed by Morse, et al[36] who found that granulocyte transfusions with a major ABO incompatibility had a lower posttransfusion recovery and survival than ABO compatible transfusions. In addition, Graw, et al[15] have shown that the posttransfusion recovery of HL-A identical, ABO incompatible granulocytes is much lower than HL-A identical, ABO compatible transfusions. Therefore, all granulocyte transfusions should be ABO compatible. When a minor incompatibility exists, excess plasma should be removed if the cells were collected by CFC. If the cells were collected by FL, there is no need to remove the supernatant solution as the amount of ABO antibody is quite small.

Rh antigens are not present on granulocytes.[34] However, the recipient may become sensitized to the $Rh_0(D)$ antigen from the red cell contamination of the granulocyte concentrate. The risk of forming anti $Rh_0(D)$ seems outweighed by the risk of sepsis in a leukopenic patient with a malignant disease. Thus, if it is unlikely that the patient will ever become pregnant, we would transfuse granulocytes without regard to Rh type. In practice, it is almost always possible to find an Rh compatible donor. We have administered over 500 granulocyte transfusions during the last 3½ years and not one of these has been Rh incompatible.

The importance of the HL-A system in donor selection will be discussed in Section VII in relation to recovery of transfused granulocytes. Regardless of the HL-A type, donor granulocytes and red cells must be compatible with the recipient's serum (Section VI).

IV. Effects of leukapheresis on donors

Donor reactions to FL or CFC leukapheresis are uncommon; however, some donors may experience anxiety, chilliness, and fatigue at the end of the procedure. With CFC leukapheresis, the hemoglobin falls during the procedure by 0.67 — 1.2 gms/100 ml, while the leukocyte count remains unchanged.[14,28] The platelet count decreases

30-50,000/mm³ and coagulation tests will be abnormal depending upon the anticoagulants used. We[28] found no change in total proteins, BUN, glucose, phosphorus, Na, K, Cl, CO_2, haptoglobin, plasma hemoglobin and urinalysis. Our donors experience a mild but consistent fall in total calcium (0.7 mg/100 ml) as a result of CFC leukapheresis, although none experienced symptoms suggestive of hypocalcemia. Graw, et al[14] found no abnormality in renal and liver function when donors were followed for up to 24 months.

Herzig, et al[17] found an average hemoglobin loss of 0.85 gm/100 ml, and the average platelet loss was 39,000/mm³ in 17 donors who underwent 33 filtration leukaphereses. There was no change in blood chemistries, hepatic and renal function although specific tests performed and specific results were not reported. Djerassi[16] found that in six donors studied, FL did not alter calcium, glucose, bicarbonate, haptoglobin, bilirubin, SGOT, and total protein. Hematocrit, leukocyte count, and platelet count were essentially unchanged two to seven days after FL, although values immediately following leukapheresis were not reported. Djerassi, et al,[16] as well as Herzig, et al,[17] reported that some donors experienced a chilliness although this was alleviated by blankets to warm the donor. Use of a blood warmer in the FL or CFC system does not seem warranted and chilling has not been a problem in our donors undergoing either FL or CFC leukapheresis.

There appears to be a granulocytosis during FL which does not occur during CFC leukapheresis.[6,17] We have found an increase in the absolute granulocyte count in 33 of 43 FL procedures performed on 25 different donors. The mean increase in granulocyte levels in our donors was 35%. Herzig, et al[17] noted a 120% increase in granulocyte count which was sustained for approximately one hour. This FL granulocytosis seems to be associated with a plasma factor as Herzig et al[17] were able to reproduce the granulocytosis by infusing autologous plasma collected during FL.

In summary, there is rather extensive data available to indicate that the effect of leukapheresis on normal donors is minor. If leukapheresis becomes a widely used procedure, it will be necessary to establish more definite standards of donor acceptability, particularly for donors undergoing multiple leukaphereses. This will be difficult since many of these donors may be the only suitable donors available for a particular patient.

V. Function of granulocytes collected by CFC and FL

Granulocytes collected by CFC leukapheresis "appear viable by both phase and light microscopy and retained the ability to ingest latex particles."[4] We have shown that immediately after collection CFC granulocytes have normal bactericidal activity and normal ability to reduce NBT dye.[27]

Djerassi[6] reported that up to 97% of FL granulocytes were potentially viable when measured by trypan blue dye exclusion, and that 76% of the granulocytes would phagocytize yeast cells. Buchholz[2] reported that 97% of FL granulocytes were viable by trypan blue dye exclusion and that they were capable of *in vitro* bactericidal and phagocytic activity. However, Herzig, et al[17] reported decreased viability by trypan blue dye exclusion of FL granulocytes compared with a peripheral blood control. Phase miscroscopy showed marked cytoplasmic vacuolization in 15-20% of the FL granulocytes. Both phagocytic and bactericidal activity were reduced 20%.

Granulocytes collected by CFC and FL have been observed morphologically and tested for *in vitro* function in our laboratory. Granulocytes collected by CFC leukapheresis appeared morphologically normal by light microscopy. Approximately 3% of the granulocytes had increased vacuolization and an additional 8% of the cells were unrecognizable (Table 3). In contrast, 23% of FL granulocytes had

TABLE 3: Morphologic Appearance of Leukocytes Collected by FL and CFC Leukapheresis

	CFC	FL
Granulocytes		
Normal	63	61
Increased vacuolization	3	23
Unrecognizable cells	8	13
Lymphocytes	26	3
	100%	100%

increased vacuolization and 13% were unrecognizable. Using the bactericidal assay, quantitative NBT test,[29] oxygen consumption[19] and chemotaxis assay,[31] CFC granulocytes showed activity equal to granulocytes collected directly from the donor immediately before and immediately after leukapheresis, and granulocytes freshly collected in CPD from normal blood bank donors (Table 4). FL granulocytes,

TABLE 4: Function of Granulocytes Collected by CFC and FL

	Bactericidal Assay % Killing at 2 hrs. CFC	FL	Chemotaxis Assay # Cells/10 HPF CFC	FL
Donor before	87	76	191	172
Granulocyte Concentrate	87	64	222	179
Donor after	85	80	183	173
CPD Control	86	81	187	167

however, had significantly decreased bactericidal activity, killing only 64% of the bacteria in the assay. Both CFC and FL granulocytes had normal in *vitro* function when tested by the chemotaxis assay (Table 4) and the quantitative NBT test, and oxygen consumption (Table 5).

TABLE 5: Function of Granulocytes collected by CFC and FL

	NBT Assay Δ OD CFC	FL	Oxygen Consumption Microliters/hr CFC	FL
Donor before		.124		
Granulocyte Concentrate	.114	.142	8.37	10.11
Donor after		.129		
CPD Control	.113	.123	6.95	8.65

Since phagocytosis is a membrane dependent phenomenon, it is quite likely that adherence of granulocytes to nylon fibers causes damage sufficient to interfere with this process. However, we would expect to see impaired chemotactic response in that case. Further studies are underway in our laboratory to attempt to clarify this apparent inconsistency. The clinical *in vivo* significance of this mild but consistent decrease in bactericidal activity remains to be established.

VI. Posttransfusion recovery and survival of granulocytes

Much of the data concerning the effects of granulocyte transfusion on the recipient's peripheral leukocyte count and the recovery and survival of transfused granulocytes is based on transfusions of CML cells. These results should be extrapolated to normals with caution since it is not established whether the fate of CML cells is identical to that of normal cells. In evaluating the posttransfusion response, one should be certain of the terminology being used, and distinguish between posttransfusion "recovery" and "increment." The percent increment in recipient's leukocyte count is:

$$\% \text{ Increment} = \frac{(\text{posttransfusion WBC}) - (\text{pretransfusion WBC})}{\text{pretransfusion WBC}} \times 100$$

Thus, if the granulocyte count is increased from 100 pre- to 200 posttransfusion, this would be reported as a 100% increment—a figure which sounds much more impressive than the actual changes in the recipient's granulocyte count. It is also necessary to identify whether changes are reported in total leukocyte or absolute granulocyte counts.

Another method expressing the posttransfusion increment involves standardizing the dose of granulocytes transfused ($\times 10^{10}$) and the size of the patient (M^2 body surface).

$$\text{Corrected Increment} = \frac{\text{Observed granulocyte increment (mm}^3\text{)}}{\text{Total number granulocytes transfused} \times 10^{10}} \times \text{Surface area (M}^2\text{)}$$

An uncorrected increment is meaningless since it does not account for variations in the number of cells transfused or in the size of the patient.

Posttransfusion recovery of granulocytes is also expressed as a percent and should not be confused with percent increment in peripheral granulocyte levels. The posttransfusion recovery must take into account the recipient's blood volume which can be estimated based upon the surface area (2500 ml $\times M^2$) or the body weight (70 ml $\times$ kg).

We prefer to use surface area and calculate posttransfusion recovery based upon the following formula:

$$\text{\% granulocyte recovery} = \frac{(\text{Observed gran. increment/mm}^3) \times (1000) \times (\text{blood volume*})}{\text{Total number granulocytes transfused}} \times 100$$
* blood volume = body surface area (M^2) $\times$ 2500 ml

Freireich, et al[9] obtained a median increment of $1000/M^2/10^{10}$ cells transfused resulting from transfusion of a median of 5.8×10^{10} CML granulocytes. The percent of transfused CML cells recovered in the recipient's circulation depended upon the initial granulocyte level, and ranged from 2% in patients with absolute granulocyte counts $< 10/mm^3$ up to 7.5% in patients with absolute granulocyte counts $> 1000/mm.^3$

Morse, et al[36] reported a median granulocyte increment of 1,000 when a median of 6.8×10^{10} CML granulocytes were transfused. It is not clear whether this is an observed or corrected increment. The median posttransfusion recovery was 4.8% and also varied from 2.1%—8.6%, depending upon the patient's initial granulocyte level.

Goldstein, et al[10] studied 78 transfusions of CML granulocytes to 34 patients with acute leukemia. The median number of cells transfused was 2×10^{10} which produced a median increment (corrected) of 220/mm^3 and a 5.5% recovery. However, some of these recipients had circulating leukocyte antibodies which made the transfusions incompatible.

Eyre, et al[8] studied transfusion of CML granulocytes into four patients with acute leukemia. Posttransfusion recovery was 19% and 49% in the two patients without circulating leukocyte antibody after infusion of approximately 2×10^{10} CML cells.

Graw, et al[12] reported median recovery of 15% of CML granulocytes transfused into recipients who did not have circulating leukocyte antibody. In an earlier report,[11] these investigators obtained a median increment (not corrected) of 1400/mm^3 when 1×10^{11} CML granulocytes were transfused, and 600 when 1×10^{10} normal granulocytes were transfused. It was suggested that higher posttransfusion increments can be obtained from an equivalent number of normal cells compared with CML cells. In a separate report, Graw, et al[15] obtained a corrected posttransfusion corrected increment of 850/mm^3 when 0.56×10^{10} normal granulocytes collected by CFC were transfused.

Thus, to summarize, almost all of the data currently available in published, documented form concerns transfusion of CML granulocytes. Most investigators report that 5-10% of CML granulocytes transfused to patients with acute leukemia can be recovered in the circulation one hour after transfusion. However, all of these patients have extremely low granulocyte levels prior to transfusion, and the data should be judged with the accuracy of leukocyte counting at these levels in mind. Posttransfusion recoveries and increments probably are different for normal compared with CML granulocytes.

All of the above data refers to granulocytes collected either by conventional plastic bag leukapheresis or by CFC leukapheresis. There is very little data concerning posttransfusion recovery and survival of granulocytes collected by FL. Graw, et al[15] found that although the number of granulocytes collected by FL was almost four times that of CFC leukapheresis (20.4 versus 5.6×10^9), the corrected posttransfusion increment in granulocyte count was smaller in transfusions of FL cells (233 versus 850/mm^3). As further evidence of the shortened intravascular survival of FL granulocytes, the one hour posttransfusion increment was significantly smaller for FL compared with CFC granulocytes when cells were collected by both methods in the same donor recipient pair.[17] The intravascular survival (DFP^{32} half life) of granulocytes collected from dogs by FL was 1.25 hours compared with six hours for granulocytes collected by CFC.[17] I am not aware of any other reports of measurements of intravascular survivial of FL granulocytes, or a comparison of posttransfusion increments of FL and CFC granulocytes. Data currently available suggest that although more granulocytes can be collected by FL than CFC, these cells have a decreased recovery and short survival. Whether CFC and FL granulocytes will have equal *in vivo* effectiveness in controlling infection in leukopenic patients remains to be demonstrated.

VII. Compatibility testing for granulocyte transfusion

Compatibility testing of granulocyte concentrates should be performed using both red cell and leukocyte techniques. Red cell compatibility testing should include saline room temperature, albumin 37° and antiglobulin phases. Although segments are ideal for most compatibility testing, the large number of leukocytes in the granulocyte concentrate segment may interfere with red cell testing. Granulocytes' natural tendency to adhere may cause a false positive red cell crossmatch; however, this will not appear the same as true red cell agglutination to an experienced technologist. In addition, a leukoagglutinin may be detected occasionally in the room temperature phase of the red cell crossmatch if cells from the segment are used. Therefore, red cell compatibility testing should be performed from a pilot tube instead of segments. Eyre, et al[8] demonstrated a decreased posttransfusion recovery of granulocytes when incompatibility was demonstrated by leukoagglutination. In addition, these compatible granulocytes had a very short intravascular half life, were sequestered in the spleen, and did not localize in sites of infection in the recipient. Graw, et al[12] have shown that the recovery of CML granulocytes one hour after transfusion is 0% if there are circulating leukocyte antibodies directed against donor cells. When the donor leukocytes are compatible by lymphocytotoxicity (LC) and leukoagglutination (LA), posttransfusion recoveries ranged from 5%—24% with a median of 15%.

Goldstein, et al[10] found posttransfusion corrected increments of 360/mm³ in recipients without circulating leukocyte antibodies and 0/mm³ in patients with antibodies. Similarly, the one hour posttransfusion recovery resulting from these CML granulocytes was 9.1% for patients without leukocyte antibodies and 0% in patients with antibodies. In three patients with leukocyte antibodies directed against some but not all donors, transfusion of granulocytes compatible by

LC and LA resulted in normal posttransfusion increments and recoveries.

In addition to poor posttransfusion recoveries when leukocyte incompatibility exists between donor and recipient, HL-A similarity appears to be important. Graw, et al[12] have shown that in patients without circulating leukocyte antibodies, the recovery of granulocytes one hour following transfusion ranges from 24% in HL-A identical donor recipient pairs to 5.5% in pairs with three or more HL-A antigen differences. McCredie, et al[25] reported that the "percent increment" in peripheral granulocyte count ranged from 40% for identical twin transfusions to 10% for parent-child transfusions. Koza, et al[22] found that eight of nine patients who received granulocyte transfusions with one or no mismatch survived infection, while only 5 of 10 survived when two or more mismatches were present. In a separate report, Graw, et al[15] observed granulocyte recoveries which ranged from 50% to 3% depending upon the number of HL-A mismatches present.

The exact methods for detecting all clinically significant WBC antibodies are not known. LC has gained widespread acceptance because of its apparent relevance to organ transplantation, and because it is standardized, reproducible, and test cells can be frozen. However, we have shown that agglutination techniques have more clinical significance in the investigation of febrile transfusion reactions.[30] Granulocyte compatibility testing should be performed using lymphocytotoxicity or leukoagglutination, or both. However, further studies should be undertaken to evaluate granulocyte recovery and survival *in vivo* in relation to *in vitro* compatibility in various systems, so that a standardized system can be developed such as exists for red cell transfusion. This will undoubtedly require further refinement and development of new techniques, since clinical reactions and poor recoveries occur despite apparent compatibility using existing techniques.

VIII. Patient clinical reactions

Buckner[4] reported that the majority of recipients of granulocytes collected by CFC experienced a sharp rise in temperature and/or chills shortly following transfusion of CML granulocytes. Morse, et al[36] observed a temperature spike in 67% of afebrile patients who received transfusions of granulocytes collected by plastic bag leukapheresis from CML donors. Eyre, et al[8] observed chills, fever and malaise in two recipients who received granulocytes with incompatibility demonstrated by leukoagglutination. These cells were collected by CFC from CML donors. Goldstein, et al[10] found that 19 of 21 transfusions (90%) to patients with preformed leukocyte antibodies were associated with clinical reactions, while only 11% of 57 transfusions to patients without leukocyte antibodies were associated with reactions. These cells were also collected by CFC from CML donors. On the contrary, Koza, et al[22] reported that adverse reactions to transfusion of CFC granulocytes were uncommon. Graw, et al[15] observed no clinical reactions following transfusion of compatible granulocytes collected by CFC from normal donors, but did observe that most patients receiving compatible granulocytes collected by FL experienced chills and fever.

We have observed febrile reactions in some patients who have received granulocytes collected from normal donors by CFC which were compatible *in vitro* by lymphocytotoxicity and leukoagglutination. On the other hand, we have transfused normal granulocytes collected by CFC which were incompatible by LC and LA with no clinical reaction whatsoever. Despite the absence of clinical reaction, transfusion of incompatible granulocytes may be quite hazardous since Graw, et al[11] have shown a further loss of previously circulating leukocytes.

The lack of predictability of clinical reactions indicates that present compatibility testing methods for granulocyte transfusions are not satisfactory. Despite LC and LA compatibility testing, some transfusions will result in febrile reactions. Whether these reactions are more frequent from FL than CFC granulocytes remains to be established.

Additional complications of granulocyte transfusion are similar to other blood products. Red cell hemolysis, hepatitis, congestive heart failure, allergic reactions, malaria, and even toxoplasmosis has been reported.

Although many patients who receive granulocyte transfusions are immunosuppressed, the possibility of sensitization to leukocyte antigens must be considered. We have studied the development of leukocyte antibodies following granulocyte transfusion in 36 patients of whom 31 had acute leukemia, 3 lymphoma and 2 aplastic anemia.[40] Ten of the 36 patients developed leukocyte antibodies, and all but one of these developed before the fifth transfusion. Thus it appears that up to 25% of patients receiving granulocyte transfusions may develop leukocyte antibodies and those patients who develop antibodies are likely to do so early in the course of transfusion therapy. Prophylactic granulocyte transfusion may result in the patient becoming sensitized before granulocytes and platelets are needed to manage a specific infectious or bleeding episode.

In this small series of 31 patients the risk of developing leukocyte antibodies was related to the HL-A similarity between donor and recipient (Table 6). Leukocyte antibodies did not develop in the

TABLE 6: Influence of HL-A Matching on Leukocyte Antibody Formation*

	Total Number of Patients	Number of Patients Sensitized	% Sensitized
Mixture of Related Donors	14	3	21
Single Related Donors	16	6	37
HL-A Identical	1	0	0
1 Haplotype Mismatch	12	4	33
2 Haplotype Mismatch	3	2	67

* From Wood, N.E., D. Hadlock, J. McCullough and E.J. Yunis; Leukocyte Antibodies following Leukocyte Transfusion, **Transfusion** 13: 353, 1973 (abstract).

patient who received granulocyte transfusions from an HL-A identical sibling while 33% of the patients who received transfusions from a donor with one haplotype mismatch developed antibodies and 67% of the patients who received cells mismatched at both haplotypes developed antibodies.

One complication unique to granulocyte transfusion is graft-versus-host (GVH) reaction. Djerassi, et al[7] observed bone marrow changes, rash, diarrhea and unexplained fever in 5 of 52 patients who received transfusions of FL granulocytes obtained from normal donors. The syndrome was compatible with, but not necessarily diagnostic of GVH. Graw et al[13] reported a fatal case of GVH in a bone marrow transplant patient who received CML granulocyte transfusions. Schwarzenberg, et al[38] reported 9 cases of GVH in 46 patients who received transfusions of CML granulocytes. The patients' diagnoses consisted primarily of acute leukemia but included Hodgkins disease, aplastic anemia and CLL. The risk of GVH was directly related to the number of granulocytes transfused.

Although the possibility of GVH must be considered following granulocyte transfusions, it appears much more likely following transfusion of CML cells than normal cells. This may be due to the larger number of cells transfused and possibly because of the malignant nature of the more immature cells present. It has been suggested that irradiation of the granulocyte concentrate prior to transfusion will prevent GVH.[20] We do not feel that it is necessary to irradiate granulocyte concentrates obtained from normal donors unless the transfusions are for patients with a congenital immunodeficiency or patients undergoing bone marrow transplantation.

IX. Clinical value of granulocyte transfusions

Evaluation of the efficacy of granulocyte transfusion suffers from a paucity of thorough, well-controlled studies. One of the major problems is the selection of proper clinical criteria to evaluate. One can measure the response of the granulocyte count, or improvement in temperature, but attempts to quantitate recovery from the infectious episode, length of hospital stay, over-all survival, or remission in acute leukemia are much more difficult. In 1965, Freireich, et al[9] reported that 54% of the recipients of 80 CML transfusions experienced a return of temperature to normal. The larger the number of cells transfused, the more likely the temperature improvement. Doses of CML granulocytes less than 1×10^{10} rarely were effective in reducing fever. Morse, et al[36] also found that 54% of 81 febrile patients had normalization of their temperature following transfusion of CML granulocytes. Schwarzenberg, et al[38] noted that 50% of 48 patients had a "good response" to the transfusion of CML granulocytes. A good response was defined as either disappearance of fever or increase in leukocyte count. All of the above studies concern transfusion of granulocytes collected from CML patients.

Djerassi, et al[7] administered 654 transfusions to 52 leukopenic patients. Seven patients who received more than 10 transfusions were described in detail. All seven recovered from "apparent septic infections" although only three of the patients had positive blood cultures.

Koza, et al[22] obtained 70% recovery from infection in 20 leukopenic patients with either suspected or proven infection.

McCredie, et al[25] reported clinical results of 285 granulocyte transfusions from normal donors to 73 febrile leukopenic patients. Response was determined by "objective signs and clinical improvement as measured by conversion of positive cultures . . . lysis of fever and the clearing of infected lesions or the resolution of infiltrates on chest X-ray." Based upon these criteria, 64% of the patients responded. The median survival of the responders was 22 weeks compared with two weeks in the "nonresponders." No nontransfused infected control group was studied.

Schiffer, et al[39] found "definite clinical improvement" in three patients, "stabilization" of the infection in nine patients, and progression of the infection in eight patients who received transfusions of FL granulocytes. Thus, there were positive clinical effects in 12 of 20 (60%) patients.

Graw, et al[15] carried out controlled clinical trials of granulocyte transfusion. Thirty-nine patients with acute leukemia, aplastic anemia, or solid tumors who had an absolute granulocyte count $<500/mm^3$ and documented gram negative sepsis, received 96 granulocyte transfusions from normal donors. A nontransfused control group consisted of patients with similar diagnoses, granulocyte levels and sepsis. Approximately 30% of the control group survived the episode of gram negative sepsis while 46% of the transfused group survived. This difference is not statistically significant; however, when only patients who received four or more transfusions were compared with controls, differences in survival (100% versus 26%) are statistically significant.

Higby, et al[18] also reported a controlled trial of granulocyte transfusion in infected neutropenic leukemic patients. Granulocytes were collected from normal donors by FL. Seven of eight patients in the transfused group became afebrile by day 10 and eight of nine were alive by day 20. In the control group, three of 10 were afebrile by day 10 and three survived to day 20.

We have studied 98 granulocyte transfusions from related normal donors to 17 patients with acute nonlymphocytic leukemia who had 23 febrile episodes. Retrospective pair matching was used to established a control group of 22 patients who experienced 35 febrile episodes. We were unable to demonstrate any significant difference in the length of the febrile episode, fever during 24 hours following transfusion, survival from the febrile episode, or clearing of infection. Although it is possible that these results are due to an insufficient number of granulocytes transfused, these patients received approximately the same number of granulocytes as reported by Graw, et al.[15] Approximately 70% of the patients in our series who received granulocyte transfusions survived the febrile episode; a figure similar to that reported by Koza, et al[22] and McCredie, et al.[25] However, 76% of the nontransfused control group survived in our series, thus making the benefits of granulocyte transfusion unclear. Further well-controlled clinical trials of granulocyte transfusion are indicated to establish the therapeutic indications, and to evaluate the clinical effectiveness of cells collected by different methods.

X. Granulocyte Preservation

Although it has been considered that granulocytes remain functional for only a few hours after collection into citrate anticoagulants, we have shown that granulocytes collected by phlebotomy into plastic bags retain normal bactericidal activity, NBT activity, and nearly normal chemotactic response [26, 29, 31] after 18-24 hours storage at 4 C. Since granulocytes for transfusion are not collected by conventional phlebotomy as in these studies, the effects of storage on CFC and FL collected granulocytes were evaluated. At least 10 granulocyte concentrates collected by CFC and FL were tested using four different assays. Neither the quantitative NBT test nor the oxygen consumption assay showed a change in activity of FL granulocytes following 24 hours of storage. However, CFC granulocytes showed a decrease in the oxygen consumption assay after 24 hours storage (Table 7).

TABLE 7: Function of Granulocytes collected by FL and CFC Leukapheresis and stored for 24 hours at 4 C.

	NBT Assay Δ OD CFC	NBT Assay Δ OD FL	Oxygen Consumption Micoliters O₂/hr CFC	Oxygen Consumption Micoliters O₂/hr FL
FRESH Granulocyte Concentrate	.114	.142	8.64	10.11
CPD Control	.113	.123	7.99	8.65
STORED Granulocyte Concentrate	.120	.132	5.59	9.60
CPD Control	.119	.116	8.82	9.18

Granulocytes collected by FL had slightly impaired bactericidal activity immediately after collection and this was severely decreased following storage (Table 8). Bactericidal activity of CFC granulocytes remained normal while the chemotactic response of both CFC and FL granulocytes was impaired after 24 hours of storage.

TABLE 8: Function of Granulocytes collected by FL and CFC Leukapheresis and stored for 24 hours at 4C.

	Bactericidal Assay % Killing at 2 hrs. CFC	Bactericidal Assay % Killing at 2 hrs. FL	Chemotaxis Assay # Cells/10 HPF CFC	Chemotaxis Assay # Cells/10 HPF FL
FRESH Granulocyte Concentrate	87	64	226	195
CPD Control	86	76	201	196
STORED Granulocyte Concentrate	86	14	90	114
CPD Control	84	78	193	173

Using eosin dye exclusion, Djerassi[6] found approximately a 25% loss of viability of FL granulocytes after 24 hours of storage at 4 C. There was approximately 30% loss of viability of FL granulocytes after 24 hours when tested by a yeast phagocytosis technique. Schiffer, et al[39] reported that granulocyte viability was maintained during 24-hour storage at room temperature.

These preliminary *in vitro* data suggest that granulocytes may remain functional for up to 24 hours after collection. Preliminary studies indicate that the posttransfusion recovery and survival of stored granulocytes are normal.[27]

Further studies, however, are required. In addition, the clinical value of stored granulocytes must be established. Since *in vivo* functional data are not presently available, granulocytes should be administered as soon as possible after collection. However, transfusion of stored granulocytes may be more practical than previously believed.

The studies in this report attributed to the University of Minnesota involved many persons in addition to the author. Specific recognition should go to Drs. Ignacio Fortuny, Edmond Yunis, Daniel Hadlock, Amos Deinard, Clara Blomfield, Mark Nesbitt, William Krivit, Paul Quie, and Ms. Judy Smith, Ann Lillehaugen, Barbara Weiblen and Nancy Wood.

REFERENCES

1. Bodey GP, Buckley M, Sathe YS, et al: Quantitative relationships between circulating leukocytes and infection in patients with acute leukemia. *Ann. Int. Med.* **64**:328, 1966.

2. Buchholz DH, Wiernik PH, Mardiney MR: Granulocyte procurement by leukocyte filtration. AABB-ISBT International Transfusion Congress 1972 (abstract).

3. Buchholz DH, Schiffer CA, Wiernik PH, et al: Description and evaluation of a low cost system for filtration leukapheresis. *Transfusion* **13**:354, 1973 (abstract).

4. Buckner D, Graw RG, Eisel RJ, et al: Leukapheresis by continuous flow centrifugation (CFC) in patients with chronic myelocytic leukemia (CML). *Blood* **33**:353, 1969.

5. Djerassi I, Kim JS, Mitrakul C, et al: Filtration leukapheresis for separation and concentration of transfusable amounts of normal human granulocytes. *J. Med. (Basel)* **1**:358, 1970.

6. Djerassi I, Kim JS, Suvansri U, et al: Continuous flow flltration leukapheresis. *Transfusion* **12**:75, 1972.

7. Djerassi I, Kim J, Suvansri U: Clinical effects of massive transfusions of normal granulocytes separated by filtration leukapheresis. AABB-ISBT International Transfusion Congress 1972 (abstract).

8. Eyre HJ, Goldstein IM, Perry S, et al: Leukocyte transfusions: Function of transfused granulocytes from donors with chronic myelocytic leukemia. *Blood* **36**:432, 1970.

9. Freireich EJ, Levin RH, Whang J, et al: The Function and fate of transfused leukocytes from donors with chronic myelocytic leukemia in leukopenic recipients. *Ann. N.Y. Acad. Sci.* **113**:1081, 1965.

10. Goldstein IM, Eyre HJ, Terasaki PI, et al: Leukocyte transfusions: Role of leukocyte alloantibodies in determining transfusion response. *Transfusion* **11**:19, 1971.

11. Graw RG, Henderson ES, Perry S: Leukocyte procurement and transfusion into leukopenic patients. *Colloques Internationaux du Centre National de la Recherche Scientifique No. 185,* 1970.

12. Graw RG, Goldstein IM, Eyre HJ, et al: Histocompatibility testing for leucocyte transfusion. *Lancet* **ii**:77, 1970.

13. Graw RG, Buckner CD, Whang-Peng J, et al: Complication of bone marrow transplantation: Graft-versus-Host disease resulting from chronic myelogenous leukemia leucocyte transfusions. *Lancet* **ii**:338, 1970.

14. Graw RG, Herzig GP, Eisel RJ, et al: Leukocyte and platelet collection from normal donors with the continuous flow blood cell separator. *Transfusion* **11**:94, 1971.

15. Graw RG, Herzig G, Perry S, et al: Normal Granulocyte trans fusion therapy: Treatment of septicemia due to gram-negative bacteria. *New Eng. J. Med.* **287**:367, 1972.

16. Hersh EM, Bodey GP, Nies BA, et al: Causes of death in acute leukemia. *JAMA* **193**:105, 1965.

17. Herzig G, Root RK, Graw RG: Granulocyte collection by continuous flow filtration leukapheresis. *Blood* **39**:554, 1972.

18. Higby DJ, Henderson ES, Holland JF: Granulocyte transfusion therapy: Clinical and laboratory studies. Proceedings of AACR and ASCO, 1974 (abstract).

19. Holmes B, Page AR, Good RA: Studies of metabolic activity of leukocytes and patients with genetic abnormality of phagocytic function. *J. Clin. Invest.* **46**:1422, 1967.

20. Hong R, Gatti RA, Good RA: Hazards and potential benefits of blood transfusion in immunological deficiency. *Lancet* **ii**:388, 1968.
21. Huestis D: Personal communication, 1974.
22. Koza I, Holland JF, Cohen E: Histocompatible leukocyte transfusions during granulocytopenia. *Neoplasma* **18**:185, 1971.
23. Levine AS, Graw RG, Young RC: Management of infections in patients with leukemia and lymphoma: Current concepts and experimental approaches. *Sem. Hematol.* **9**:141, 1972.
24. McCredie KB, Freireich EJ: The Use of etiocholanolone to increase collection of granulocytes with the IBM blood cell separator. *J.C.I.* **49**:63a, 1970 (abstract).
25. McCredie KB, Freireich EJ, Hester JP, et al: Leukocyte transfusion therapy for patients with host-defense failure. *Transplantation Proc.* **5**:1285, 1973.
26. McCullough J, Benson SJ, Yunis EJ, et al: Effect of blood bank storage on leucocyte function. *Lancet* **ii**:1333, 1969.
27. McCullough J, Weiblen B, Hadlock D, et al: *In Vitro* function and *In Vivo* survival of fresh and stored granulocytes collected using the continuous flow centrifuge. *Transfusion* **13**:354, 1973 (abstract).
28. McCullough J, Forunty IE: Laboratory evaluation of normal donors undergoing leukapheresis on the continuous flow centrifuge. *Transfusion* **13**:394, 1973.
29. McCullough J, Carter SJ, Quie PG: Effects of anticoagulants and storage on granulocyte function in bank blood. *Blood* **43**:207, 1974.
30. McCullough J, Burke ME, Wood N, et al: Microcapillary agglutination for the detection of leukocyte antibodies: Evaluation of the method and clinical significance in transfusion reactions. *Transfusion,* in press.
31. McCullough J, Weiblen BJ, Quie PG: Chemotactic activity of human granulocytes preserved in various anticoagulants. *J. Lab. Clin. Med.,* in press.
32. Mishler JM, Hadlock D, McCullough J, et al: Increased efficiency of leukocyte collection by the addition of hydroxyethyl starch to the continuous flow centrifuge. *Blood,* in press.
33. Mollison PL: *Blood Transfusion in Clinical Medicine.* Blackwell Scientific Publications, 1972, p. 230.
34. *ibid.* p. 275.

35. Morse EE, Carbone PP, Freireich EJ, et al: Repeated leukapheresis of patients with chronic myelocytic leukemia. *Transfusion* **6**:175, 1966.
36. Morse EE, Freireich EJ, Carbone PP, et al: The transfusion of leukocytes from donors with chronic myelocytic leukemia to patients with leukopenia. *Transfusion* **6**:183, 1966.
37. Nusbacher J, MacPherson JL, Manejios, et al: Leukapheresis: The effect of a single high-oral does of prednisone on granulocyte mobilization, yield and function. *Transfusion* **13**:366, 1973 (abstract).
38. Schwarzenberg L, Mothe G, Amiel JL, et al: Study of factors determining the usefulness and complications of leukocyte transfusions. *Am. J. Med.* **43**:206, 1967.
39. Schiffer C, Buchholz DH, Wiernik PH: Transfusion of granulocytes obtained by filtration leukopheresis. Proceedings of AACR and ASCO, 1974 (abstract).

FRESH BLOOD: FACT AND FANCY
Douglas W. Huestis

ALL TOO OFTEN, there is something about a request for "fresh blood" that brings out the worst in both the requesting physician and the blood bank. The physician often is thinking in vague terms about an unclear clinical requirement, and has the feeling that the desired property of blood is most likely labile under storage. The more unsure he is, the more he may resent the blood bank's questioning his order. On the other hand, the blood bank often dislikes the implication that their regular stored blood is not adequate. In addition, blood bank routine usually entails using the oldest blood first, and the staff is inclined to be suspicious of a request that reverses the usual order of things, even if recently collected blood is available. If convincing clinical indications are not adduced, the blood bank staff will probably leap to the conclusion that freshness is not really important.

Both attitudes are wrong.

The physician making any special request to the blood bank should know exactly what his patient needs, and whether this is indeed present in blood, stored or otherwise. His efforts are doomed to failure, for example, if he expects to transfuse a healing factor, rejuvenation hormone, vital spirits, or some other magical property that is not scientifically demonstrable in blood. In general, he would be wiser to consult a blood bank physician before making a specific request.

On the other side of the fence, the blood bank staff should not look on the request for fresh blood as an insult or a form of persecution. Rather it should be regarded as a signal for help. In essence, since no one definition of "fresh" can fit all circumstances, it is a call for consultation, though seldom so phrased. The blood bank is not a supermarket, but a medical service.

Consultative role of the blood bank

The reason behind the growing requirement for physician participation in blood bank decision-making lies in the increasing complexity of the blood bank's inventory. Since the routine use of whole blood in most situations nowadays can only be considered irresponsible, most of what the blood bank has on its shelves will be red blood cells and other components at various stages of their storage lives. This being the case, and bearing in mind that few physicians can be expected to be completely familiar with the ways in which the blood bank can meet a given clinical requirement, the active participation of a physician has become essential in both community and hospital blood banks. It is the blood bank physician's responsibility to know the changes that take place during storage of blood and components, to be able to balance these against a particular patient's needs (in consultation with the patient's own physician), and to provide rational replacement therapy with minimal disruption of the usual orderly handling of the blood bank's inventory and processing. If, at times, non-routine procedures are required, he will be able to explain the clinical background and necessity to the blood bank staff, thus avoiding morale problems.

This all involves discussion and negotiation at a clinical level, and the blood bank technical staff, no matter how competent, cannot, as a rule, effectively fulfill such a consultative function. For many reasons, good and bad, a physician is usually required.

How the good things fare in stored blood

All biologic materials deteriorate in time, depending on their innate characteristics and on the conditions of preservation. Let us review the characteristics of the desirable parts of blood as they survive in stored whole blood. We should bear in mind that the anticoagulants approved for blood collection and storage were designed, for the most part, many years ago with an eye to red blood cell preservation, and are not necessarily optimal for other items. Also, most data in the literature refer to blood stored in ACD, whereas most blood banks now use CPD. Figure 1 shows curves for the principal components of concern. References for these data are given in the following sections.

Red blood cells

The time-honored and generally accepted dictum is that mediums used for blood storage must be such as to assure a minimum of 70 percent survival of transfused red blood cells, measured 24 hours after transfusion. If blood in a given anticoagulant reaches this point at 21 days, then that is the storage period allowed. Although data have been published to show that CPD blood[12] and, less convincingly, ACD blood as well, are still above the 70 percent range even at 28 days (see Mollison,[9] pages 60-61), such data have not convinced FDA to permit storage beyond 21 days, even for CPD blood. Despite this, we can be confident that most properly stored blood is well above the

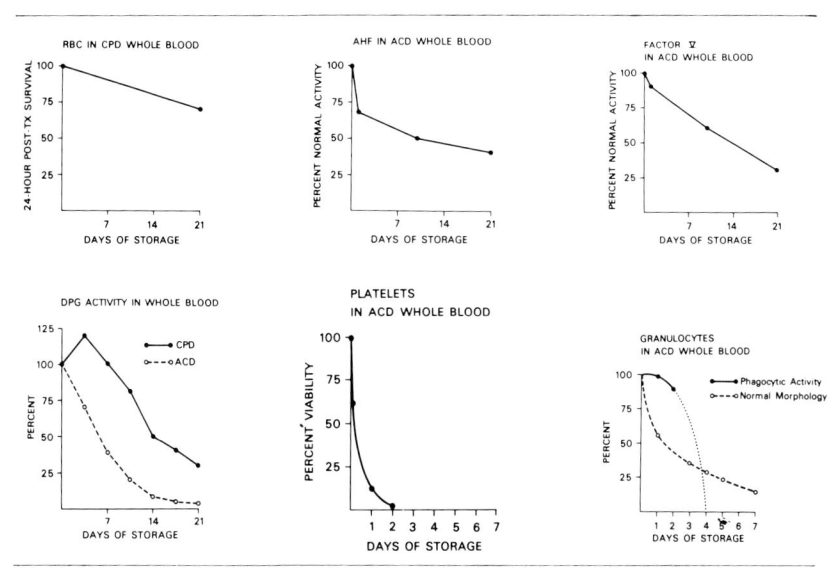

FIGURE 1

curve shown in Figure 1. Mollison[9] (page 50) has shown that red cells in ACD storage for 14 days have about 90 percent posttransfusion survival at 24 hours, which is a useful figure to remember.

DPG activity

The ability of red cell hemoglobin to release oxygen to the tissues is directly related to the cellular content of 2, 3-diphosphoglycerate (DPG). DPG decreases on blood storage, particularly in ACD, and DPG-deficient red cells tend to retain oxygen rather than releasing it. Figure 1 shows a comparison of DPG loss in ACD and CPD blood.[11] Note that the DPG level for CPD blood at 14 days is about the same as that of ACD blood at five or six days.

There have been numerous articles on DPG in stored blood, and on decreased DPG in patients who have received large amounts of stored blood, but no one has yet shown that the use of DPG-deficient blood presents a real hazard to the recipient. In fact, the history of blood transfusion is replete with instances of massive use of stored (DPG-deficient) ACD blood in the successful resuscitation of seriously injured or ill patients. Furthermore, DPG is rapidly restored in depleted red cells after transfusion (50 percent within four hours).[3] Still, DPG depletion is a theoretic hazard, and is worth considering in the selection of blood for patients in whom even a temporary restriction in oxygen delivery to the tissues might be dangerous.

Antihemophilic factor (AHF, Factor VIII)

In either ACD or CPD blood, AHF undergoes rapid attrition in the first few hours, so that roughly a third of it disappears within 24 hours of collection.[4] The remainder undergoes a much slower decay, so that after three weeks of storage there is still as much as a third of the original amount remaining. Since hemophiliacs are treated almost exclusively nowadays with AHF concentrates of one sort or another, the AHF content of stored blood is seldom a matter of concern.

Labile factor (Factor V)

Factor V does not decay as rapidly as factor VIII in the early stages, but follows a steeper overall curve, with a half life in the neighborhood of 12 days.[4,10] In considering replacement of this factor, it is important to bear in mind that 5 to 25 percent of the normal factor V is adequate for hemostasis under ordinary circumstances, although higher levels may be needed for surgical procedures or in trauma.

Platelets

Platelets are the most liable of the components ordinarily considered in transfusion. Here a sharp distinction must be made between functional viability of platelets, which is rapidly lost in whole blood storage, and countable numbers of platelets, which diminish much more slowly. The functional viability of platelets is reduced to about 12 percent by 24 hours, nearly zero by 48 hours.[2] Thus, one should not rely on whole blood or red blood cells as a source of viable platelets after about 12 hours of conventional storage.

The characteristics of platelets stored in the form of concentrates is quite a different matter, and has already been discussed in another paper.

Other clotting factors

The remainder of the clotting factors all appear to be well preserved during regular periods of blood storage.[10]

Granulocytes

Unlike lymphocytes, most of which remain viable and well preserved throughout regular blood storage, granulocytes keep their phagocytic and bactericidal capabilities for only about 48 hours, during which time they also exhibit progressive morphologic deterioration.[7] Since regular blood units, no matter how fresh, are not a practical means of transfusing granulocytes, this observation is helpful only in a negative sense.

The bad things in stored blood: how they develop

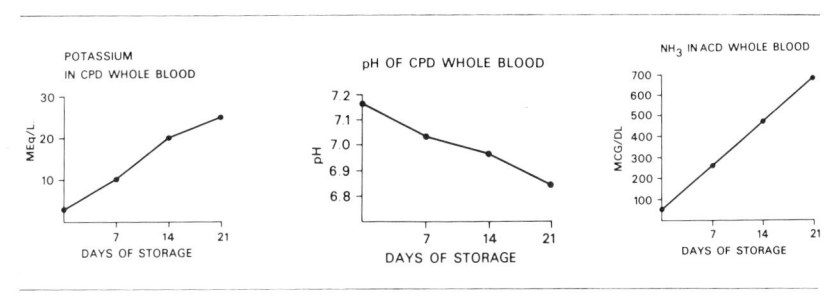

FIGURE 2

Potassium

Potassium leaks from red cells during storage in either ACD or CPD, and accumulates in the plasma. The increase is more or less rectilinear, remaining in a mild range during the first week of storage (less than 10 mEq/l in CPD blood), and is less pronounced in CPD than ACD blood. There is some evidence, mostly in experimental animals, that increased potassium aggravates the toxicity of citrate (see Mollison,[9] pages 584-586). Potassium does not ordinarily pose a serious threat except to patients whose serum potassium is already elevated (e.g., acidosis of chronic renal disease). (See Figure 2.)

Acidity

Low pH and low temperature are desirable storage conditions to maintain the viability of red blood cells, but the increasing acidity during storage (due to accumulation of lactate) may cause complications in patients with a tendency to acidosis (e.g., babies with severe hemolytic disease, or patients with chronic renal disease). In the case of CPD blood, the pH starts at a higher (more physiologic) level than

ACD, and falls gradually, but is always above the pH of ACD blood.[5] For most patients, the acidity of stored blood is of consequence only after the first week of storage. (See Figure 2.)

Ammonia

Plasma ammonia increases steadily and at a rather steep rate during blood storage.[1] There is little evidence that this poses a hazard to a recipient, except potentially in the case of severe liver failure. Ammonia levels can be considered minimal during the first week of blood storage. (See Figure 2.)

Microaggregates

Clumps of platelets, leukocytes, fibrin, and other debris form during blood storage, and have been incriminated in the cause of pulmonary vascular lesions, since they are small enough to pass through ordinary blood filters. This has been discussed extensively in another paper. Recent work indicates that at about six days of storage there is a marked increase in the filtration pressure of stored blood, this measurement being correlated with microaggregate formation.[6] See Figure 3. These data indicate that blood stored five days or less contains minimal

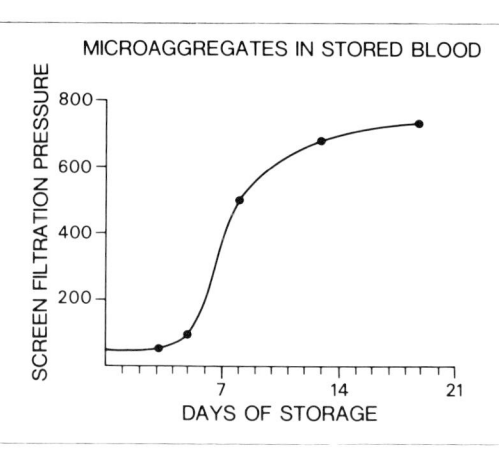

FIGURE 3

amounts of such aggregates. As a corollary, if a person is expected to receive large amounts of older stored blood, a special filter to remove microaggregates may be considered necessary.

Meeting the need

The changes in stored blood are inevitably detrimental to many of the components that make it up. Obviously, it would be best for all patients to have only fresh blood or components, were it not for the prohibitive difficulties of supplying blood in such a context, and the inherent wastefulness of not finding a use of older stored blood. In the interests of efficiency, we must compromise and decide when it is important to have a minimum of storage changes, and when a wider latitude is permissible.

In addition, almost all components can be better preserved and concentrated in smaller volume when separated from whole blood early in storage and kept under conditions optimal for that component. Most blood banks now routinely prepare and store freshly separated components, rather than waiting for special orders. Consequently, a request for immediate "fresh blood" must often be met with the reply that it is not available at the moment, but there is an inventory of freshly separated components. It is not easy to explain all this in a few moments to an anxious physician with a problem, who may find it difficult to understand why you have to "take the blood apart, then put it back together again." But the successful handling of such explanations is a primary duty of the blood bank physician today.

Some of the common clinical situations in which special patient needs may produce a request for "fresh blood" are shown in Table 1, page 124.

Massive blood replacement

When a patient's total blood volume is replaced once or twice in the course of a day with stored bank blood, the clotting factors, particularly platelets, are in effect washed out. This usually requires at least 20 units and sometimes causes a bleeding tendency with severe oozing from cut or raw surfaces. When this happens, the physician will often ask for fresh blood, and will usually be satisfied with blood within a day or two of collection. But most of these problems are caused by platelet deficiency, and blood 24 hours or more old is a poor source of platelets (see Figure 1). Unless a hemostasis evaluation reveals a more complex problem, the best solution is to provide platelet concentrates (not less than four for an adult) supplemented by bank red blood cells as needed. Red blood cells or whole blood would have to be less than 12 hours in storage to provide useful num-

TABLE 1: Requests for "Fresh Blood"

Clinical Indication	Realistic definition of "fresh" blood*	Reasonable substitutes
Bleeding due to massive blood replacement	Less than 12 h	Platelet concentrates plus RBC**; Platelet-rich RBC
Open heart surgery, before and during ECC***	Preferably less than 1 week	Bank or frozen-thawed RBC plus volume expanders
Open heart surgery, oozing after ECC	Less than 12 h	Platelet concentrates plus bank RBC; Platelet-rich RBC
Optimal red cell survival and function	Less than 1 week	Frozen-thawed RBC
Exchange transfusion	Less than 1 week	Bank or frozen-thawed RBC plus fresh plasma
Liver failure	Less than 1 week	Bank or frozen-thawed RBC plus fresh plasma
Chronic renal disease	Less than 1 week	Frozen-thawed or leukocyte-poor RBC

* Assuming CPD Red Blood Cells or Whole Blood.
** Some patients may also need fresh plasma and occasionally fibrinogen or cryoprecipitated AHF.
*** Extracorporeal circulation.

bers of platelets, and the platelets would not be concentrated, so this is not usually a practical solution.

Open heart surgery

Blood up to a week or so in storage is perfectly satisfactory for routine use to replace losses and to prime extracorporeal circuits. Older blood is usable, but may be damaged more by the pump. In fact, regular bank red blood cells, frozen-thawed red blood cells, or platelet-poor red blood cells are all satisfactory, and are used routinely at the University of Arizona. There is no need to specify whole blood for heart surgery.

If the patient is on extracorporeal circulation more than two hours, his platelet count falls, presumably because of pump damage. Oozing, as in massive transfusion washout, may then occur and require platelet concentrates. These should be reserved until after the patient is off the pump, and should not be given through one of the special filters intended to remove microaggregates. Good teamwork between the surgical group and the blood bank should permit advance notice of patients at hazard of long pump times, so that platelets will be available. Again, whole blood or platelet-rich red blood cells should be less than 12 hours stored, and are not as likely to be available.

Optimal red cell survival

For patients needing continued transfusions over long periods of time (e.g., hypoplastic anemias), to minimize the number of transfusions, iron buildup, etc., reasonably fresh red blood cells are best (such patients should never receive whole blood). For such purposes, red blood cells less than a week in storage, or frozen-thawed red blood cells are satisfactory.

Exchange transfusion

The freshest blood available should always be used for infant exchange transfusion. Nevertheless, there has been a wealth of clinical experience to indicate that ACD blood stored up to five days is satisfactory for most babies, even though we now know that it has decreased DPG content. With CPD blood now available almost everywhere, concerns over pH and DPG should fade, and CPD blood less than a week in storage should be completely satisfactory. If blood older than this is all that is available, it is probably better to remove the plasma and substitute compatible fresh-frozen plasma. This will correct the pH and potassium, but not the DPG. If the latter is a concern, then frozen-thawed red blood cells can be used with fresh plasma as an equivalent to absolutely fresh blood. Platelets are seldom necessary and can be supplied separately if needed. Any of these expedients is preferable to delaying a needed exchange transfusion while seeking "fresh blood."

Liver failure

Citrate is broken down by the normal liver, and may thus be a hazard to some patients with liver failure, particularly if exchange transfusion is being considered. Some physicians are also concerned about the ammonia content of older stored blood (see Figure 2). For exchange transfusion in fulminant hepatitis, heparinized blood is usually specified, which answers both citrate and ammonia considerations. For more routine blood replacement, bank red blood cells are satisfactory. If replacement of liver clotting factors (e.g., factor V) is necessary as well, fresh-frozen plasma may be used, supplemented as need be by bank or frozen-thawed red blood cells, or whole blood less than a week in storage. In preparation for surgical procedures, such as vascular shunts, fresh-frozen plasma can correct clotting factor deficiencies.

Chronic renal disease

For patients with chronic renal disease, it is best to avoid transfusing excess potassium, and also to provide erythrocytes that will survive optimally. Both conditions can be met by the use of red blood cells less than a week in storage. Candidates for kidney transplants should receive as few donor leukocytes as possible, to avoid immunization to HL-A antigens. This is accomplished by the use of frozen-thawed or other leukocyte-poor red blood cell preparations.

Tact, diplomacy, and consultation

By simply pointing out that the hepatitis test will not be completed, it is possible to scare off many requests for "fresh blood," but this may not be in the patient's best interest if he really needs some labile component. The request for "fresh blood" indicates a special concern for a particular patient, and the blood bank's attitude must be that of evaluating the patient's need, both qualitatively and quantitatively, and meeting it in the most expeditious way, consonant with scientific reality and operational practicality. Consequently, the approach to the patient's physician should not be a challenge ("Why do you want fresh blood?"), but rather an inquiry as to the clinical circumstances ("Tell me about your patient. . . . We have several ways of supplying blood and components and would like to see what approach would be best"). When the request specifies some property that does not exist in either fresh or stored blood, such as a healing factor, it may be necessary to point this out to the physician in a tactful way, perhaps by emphasizing the hazards of transfusion when the likely benefits are dubious. Each person must devise his own approach to this kind of situation.

Naturally, emergencies will not usually permit a leisurely approach, and the blood bank physician may have to make quick decisions based on fragmentary clinical details. As always, the proper approach is based on the desire to be helpful. This attitude on the part of the blood bank quickly becomes known to physicians and hospital departments, and does much to prevent the kind of resentment that may occur when a blood request is questioned.

This discussion by no means has been a complete exposition of the many reasons for "fresh blood" requests, nor of all the ways of handling such requests. Rather, it is intended to summarize the principal areas of legitimate clinical concern and the various alternatives open to the blood bank in each case. There are certainly other areas of reasonable concern, and even more numerous myths and fancies that can influence transfusion requests. These would make a most entertaining discussion and exchange of experience, but time does not permit the luxury. My aim has been to present the background for rational treatment of an often irrational request. Each person must take this and adapt it to circumstances and personalities as he sees best.

REFERENCES

1. *Technical Methods and Procedures,* 5th edition. Chicago, American Association of Blood Banks, 1970, p. 196.

2. Baldini M, Costea N, Dameshek W: The viability of stored human platelets. *Blood* **16**:1669, 1960.

3. Beutler E: Maintenance of red cell function during storage. *In:* AABB-ISBT Progress in Transfusion and Transplantation. Washington, D.C., AABB, 1972.

4. Bowie EJW, et al: The stability of antihemophilic factor and labile factor in human blood. *Mayo Clin. Proc.* **39**:144, 1964.

5. Dawson RB, et al: Hemoglobin functions and 2, 3-DPG levels of blood stored 4 C in ACD and CPD. pH effect. *Transfusion* **10**:299, 1970.

6. Harp JR, et al: Some factors determining rate of microaggregate formation in stored blood. *Anesthesiology* **40**:398, 1974.

7. McCullough J, et al: Effect of blood-bank storage on leucocyte function. *Lancet* **2**:1333, 1969.

8. McCullough, J, Carter SJ, Quie PG: Effects of anticoagulants and storage on granulocyte function in bank blood. *Blood* **43**:207, 1974.

9. Mollison PL: *Blood Transfusion in Clinical Medicine,* 5th edition. Oxford, Blackwell Scientific Publications, 1972.

10. Owen Jr, CA, et al: *The Diagnosis of Bleeding Disorders.* Boston, Little, Brown & Co., 1969, pages 186-193.

11. Shafer AW, et al: 2, 3-diphosphoglycerate in red cells stored in acid-citrate-dextrose and citrate-phosphate-dextrose: Implications regarding delivery of oxygen. *J. Lab. Clin. Med.* **77**:430, 1971.

12. Shields CE: Comparison studies of whole blood stored in ACD and CPD and with adenine. *Transfusion* **8**:1, 1968.